D0927465

Development Communication

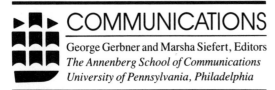

COMMUNICATIONS
George Gerbner and Marsha Siefert, Editors
The Annenberg School of Communications
University of Pennsylvania, Philadelphia

Development Communication

INFORMATION, AGRICULTURE, AND NUTRITION IN THE THIRD WORLD

ROBERT C. HORNIK

The Annenberg School of Communications
University of Pennsylvania, Philadelphia

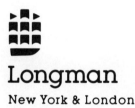

Longman

New York & London

Development Communication:
Information, Agriculture, and Nutrition in the Third World

Longman Inc., 95 Church Street, White Plains, N.Y. 10601

Associated companies:
Longman Group Ltd., London
Longman Cheshire Pty., Melbourne
Longman Paul Pty., Auckland
Copp Clark Pitman, Toronto
Pitman Publishing Inc., New York

Executive editor: Gordon T. R. Anderson
Production editors: Elsa van Bergen/Katherine Rangoon
Text design: Steven August Krastin
Cover design: Steven August Krastin
Cover illustration/photo: Steven August Krastin
Production supervisor: Eduardo Castillo

Library of Congress Cataloging-in-Publication Data

Hornik, Robert C.
    Development communication: information
agriculture and nutrition in the third world
        (Communications / the Annenberg School
of Communications, University of Pennsylvania, Philadelphia)
        1. Communication—Developing countries.
2. Communication in agriculture—Developing countries.
3. Communication of technical information—Developing
countries. I. Title. II. Series: Communications
(Annenberg School of Communications (University of
Pennsylvania))
P92.2.H67 1988   001.51'09172'4   86-27327
ISBN 0-582-28520-8

Compositor: Best-Set Typesetter, Ltd.
Printer: The Maple-Vail Book Manufacturing Group

87 88 89 90 9 8 7 6 5 4 3 2 1

Contents

Preface   ix

Part One: COMMUNICATION AND DEVELOPMENT—   1
            AN OVERVIEW

1 **The Roles of Communication in Education/Information Projects**   3

   Communication as Low-Cost Loudspeaker   3
   Communication Technology as Institutional Catalyst   5
   Communication as Political Lightning Rod   5
   Communication as Organizer and Maintainer   6
   Communication as Equalizer   7
   Communication for Improvement in Quality   8
   Communication Technology as Accelerator of Interaction   9
   Communication as Legitimator/Motivator   10
   Communication for Feedforward   10
   Communication as Magnifier of Dependency/Integration   11
   Communication Programs for Creating and Supplying Demand   12

2 **Why Communication for Development So Rarely Succeeds**   14

   Theory Failures   14
   Program Failures   17
   Political Explanation of Failure   24

Part Two: COMMUNICATION AND AGRICULTURE   27

3 **The Roles of Information in Agriculture**   29

   Information Flows to the Farmer   30
   Factor and Market Price Information   39
   Information Flows to Develop Farmer Organization   41
   Information Flows to Agricultural Technicians   42
   Information Flows from Farmers   43

4 Information Programs Without Communication Technology   47

   Conventional Extension   48
   Approaches to Resolving the Major Issues   55

5 Communication Technology for Agriculture   69

   Typical Uses of Communication Technology   69
   Improving the Utility of Communication in Agriculture   73
   Other Media-Based Information Systems   83

6 Summary and Implications: Agriculture   87

   The Roles of Information   87
   Information Programs Without Communication Technology   87
   Information Programs Based on Communication Technology   89
   Implications   90

Part Three: COMMUNICATION AND NUTRITION   95

7 The Roles of Information in Nutrition   97

   The Potential for Nutrition Education   98
   Education at the Aggregate Household Level   100
   Education Within the Household   101
   Breast Feeding Among Nonrural Women   102
   Weaning-Age Malnutrition   107
   Nutritional Treatment of Diarrhea   113

8 On the Possibility of Doing Nutrition Education   116

   A Hypothetical Conventional System and Its Flaws   117
   Solving Problems of the Conventional Model: Past Experience   118
   Education as Complement to Material Inputs   137
   Incentives for Educators and Clients   143
   Costs and Financing   145

9 Communication in Nutrition: Conclusions   148

   Restatement of Findings   148
   Implications   151

Part Four: CONCLUSIONS   153

10 Doing Communication for Development   155

    Comparing Explanations for Project Ineffectiveness   155
    Prescriptions for Doing Information for Development Well   159
    Implications for the Design of Information Programs   162
    The Chances of Realizing the Recommended Model   164

Bibliography   167

Index   177

Preface

Most efforts to use communication technology for development do not do what they are meant to do. They do not satisfy their ostensible objectives. Nonetheless, the history of communication for development can be seen, on balance, as an optimistic one. Future efforts are more likely to succeed than many past ones.

The history of communication for development can begin anywhere: with Moses at the foot of Mount Sinai; with the encouragement of public literacy to spread the faith after the invention of the printing press; or, on a less-grand scale, with the use of radios in Australia and New Zealand in the 1930s to educate the children of farmers. The conventional history, however, begins after World War II with an extraordinary political change: the movement to independence of more than half the world's nations, most of them in the Southern Hemisphere and most of them poor by all the criteria that Northern Hemisphere nations held dear. Their per capita incomes were small, their few health systems had to serve burgeoning populations, their industrial plant — the assumed engine of modernization — was nonexistent, while their people had little education and few "modern" skills. Their social organization, including political and economic institutions, and their *apparent* lack of social mobility, intellectual dynamism, and psychological openness were all seen to stand in the way of their reaching the stage of development occupied by modern Western nations.

In the years following World War II, the predominant explanation for Southern Hemisphere poverty pointed to deficits in the poor nations and their peoples. Such nations were said to be poor because they did not save and invest enough in their industrial plant to fuel a takeoff to rapid growth; they lacked entrepreneurs to organize economic change (Hagen 1962); they lacked educated and skilled populations to serve in a modern labor force and transform static social institutions.

To the extent that those deficits lay with individuals — lack of education, skills, and modern attitudes — they demanded development solutions stressing more formal education, more training for adults, and more information diffusion. Education might provide intellectual skills; it might teach new health and agricultural practices and encourage political mobilization. However, implementing education in poor countries proved to be difficult. Conventional Western educational strategies for doing these tasks through face-to-face instruction foundered on the thin supply of teachers and trained field agents and inadequate budgets to support their work.

Thus, on the one hand, influential development theorists argued that poor rates of development might be explained, in part, by deficits in knowledge and skills among people in developing countries. On the other hand, it was readily understood that programs for repairing those deficits with face-to-face instruction were implausible. This led many to argue for using the mass media, with their potential for reaching audiences otherwise beyond the reach of government resources, either as a substitute for unavailable teachers and field agents or as a complement to inadequately trained personnel. Wilbur Schramm's 1967 UNESCO-sponsored study, "Mass Media and National Development," was an influential summary of this position. Enthusiasm for the power of mass media led to the creation of hundreds of mass-media-based projects worldwide during the 1950s, 1960s, and 1970s.

There were programs to put radios and televisions in schools, to supplement the work of classroom teachers, or to take core responsibility for instruction with the classroom teachers' assistance. There were out of school programs to reach adults with basic literacy and numeracy skills, and more advanced distance-education programs at the high school and university levels.

Agriculture, the central occupation for most of the south's population, was a prime target for communication programs. Part Two of this book traces that history. There were programs to teach health and nutrition skills to people isolated from functioning health systems. They are the subject of Part Three of this book. There were communication programs to affect family-planning decisions as population control emerged as a worldwide concern, particularly in poor nations whose limited economic resoures were being absorbed by ever-increasing populations.

Communication was also used to remedy perceived deficits in political values: programs encouraged identification with the newly established nation-state; they stimulated the social mobilization needed to transform national ideologies; they were used to legitimate the political actions of national leaders or would-be leaders.

Communication and development programs flourished for good reason. They fit with the roll-up-your-sleeves-and-do-development optimism of the age after World War II and after the Marshall Plan (which was credited with revitalizing European economies). The nature of the problems presented for solution by communication projects was politically unassailable. What constituency could argue in public against enhancing agricultural productivity or improving nutrition? Whatever the internal political agendas and choices, the outward benefits to all parties involved in the funding and execution of communication projects were demonstrably to improve the quality of life. The political climate following World War II favored the investment of government and international agency funds in aid projects, and the prevailing philosophy saw information as a commodity not unlike tractors or fertilizer in effecting a peaceful cultivation of allies. Communication development projects continued to be demonstrations of good will. Their outcomes were perhaps not as politically important as their existence and initiation, both on the part of the initiator and recipient.

A general belief in the neutrality of communication technology also enhanced its attractiveness as a solution to human problems. As a carrier of information, technology was seen to extend the reach of information while bypassing the barriers of education and class. Technology was also a glamorous solution; and once a few countries had begun to use communications technology to solve problems, it became a more universally desired route for others.

The only problem was that communication for development (and, in general, all development programs) was not producing the development that had been promised. Some have argued that expectations were unrealistic to begin with and that progress was slow but present; in fact some countries (for example, Taiwan and South Korea) made great strides. However as the 1970s and 1980s progressed, there was profound disappointment in the postwar models of development. In some nations, most obviously in sub-Saharan Africa, progress was stalled. In other nations, while some members of society had joined the modern sector, many others had been left out. There were calls, particularly from those living in the Third World, to reassess earlier explanations for slow development and earlier solutions to development problems. Third World scholars asked whether the poverty of Southern Hemisphere nations was to be explained entirely by deficits in those nations. Rather, they asked, weren't exploitative economic relationships between wealthy and poor nations of equal or greater importance? The relation of elites and nonelites within developing countries was viewed in a jaundiced light as well. For many, the image of a benevolent national and international elite sharing its progress with the less fortunate was replaced by the image of substantial conflicts of interest between those parties. Hospital beds, university educations, and food subsidies for the urban residents of a poor nation meant fewer resources to benefit its rural people. Determinations made by wealthier nations about oil prices, export-import limitations, the costs of technology transfer, and interest on loans profoundly influenced the development of poorer countries but were beyond their control.

This revisionist view of development that dominated the outlook of the 1970s was coupled with changes in perspective on what communication in particular could do for development. The human deficit model that underpinned so much of communication for development was no longer credible to many. Too often, information was being thrown at problems that were defined by lack of resources, not lack of knowledge. The assumption that if only people knew more they could readily better their situation was seen to be a cruel deception. Poverty was not only the result of failures of the poor to change, but of the powerlessness of those poor to alter the political and economic structures that limited their progress. Farmers did not buy fertilizer, not because they did not know it would increase their crop yields, but because they could not obtain the credit to purchase it. The incidence of diarrheal disease would be reduced not by changes in individual practices like boiling water or hand washing but by changes in the distribution of resources like piped water and refrigeration.

This critique joined two elements. First, there was an argument that development problems were fundamentally political problems. The problem was resource and power inequity; the solution was political organization of the poor. Second, although less explicit, was a technical criticism of previous communication-for-development programs: project managers had blithely assumed that they understood the situation of their audience, knew what was best for them, and only had to tell them what to do. If their audience failed to respond, well, what could you do? Those peasants were all fatalists anyway. Thus, an element of the critique was that project managers had not done communication for development very well. These two elements of the critique, in turn, spawned two new approaches to communication for development: communication for political organization, and doing communication for development better, or "communication as complement." Together they make up the second generation of communication-for-development projects.

One set of program developers argued that previous projects rarely benefited the poor. They explained that failure in political terms: a program controlled by central authorities and not by its beneficiaries inevitably serves the needs of the central authorities. So long as the "targets" of development efforts depend on an elite's paternalistic willingness to do good, to spend resources for the benefit of the powerless, little good will be done. The answer is to be found in small-scale efforts, run for and by the beneficiaries, called *participatory programs*. These grassroots programs have been initiated in many development sectors. In the communication-for-development arena they have involved support of local media production capacity and distribution mechanisms. The materials have sometimes had a pedagogic element that addresses health or agriculture or literacy, but they have always had a "popular promotion" function of raising political awareness and stimulating political organization in poor communities.

The other set of second-generation projects has focused on doing communication for development better. All of these projects, whether in health, agriculture, or formal education, have shared certain characteristics. In a fundamental way they have accepted that communication is a limited intervention and is constrained by other forces, and they have sought to do what can be done within those boundaries. They have invested heavily in the message-development process, they have become informed about and responsive to their audiences, and they have linked media messages to material and educational actions of other institutions. Their primary task has been to understand what problems their audiences are trying to solve and what resources they have at hand or can obtain realistically, in order to arrive at a feasible strategy, including a communication element among other components.

One group, called *interactive radio projects*, has done in-school education. In the pioneer program, teaching mathematics in Nicaragua by radio in early primary grades, fourteen professionals spent one year producing the materials for a single grade. Meticulous and artful planning of the substance and style of presentations, lessons that actively involved students, and extensive classroom observation and testing all came together to produce learning substantially better than that achieved in nonradio classrooms.

A second group has worked in the health sector and is often called *social marketing projects*. It has encouraged changes in specific behavior such as using a product like oral rehydration salts to treat diarrheal disease, or adopting new practices like using weaning foods. These projects are discussed extensively in Part Three.

This is a broad outline of the joint history of development and of communication for development: Slow development was seen to be due in part to human deficits, and communication projects were created to remedy these deficits. Then, continued slow development was seen to be the consequence of national and international economic and power inequities, and communication was used for political organization or to achieve limited but valued outcomes within boundaries set by economic and political systems.

However, this history is a partial history, a simplified history, and an unfinished history. It is partial because, as a history of communication and development, it includes only the deliberate uses of communication to achieve specific development outcomes. It leaves out the evolution of mass media institutions — the press, radio, and television — insofar as they do not touch directly on the achievement of sectorial development outcomes. It ignores the flow of news and entertainment programing across national boundaries, the subject of much current writing.

It is a simplified history because it emphasizes the shifts in ideology and related practice and leaves out much of the detail and the variety. Only at the crudest level can we place all of the developing nations in the world in a single conceptual frame. And while we can talk about shifts in ideas about how communication for development should be done, those movements may hide a practice that is changing much more slowly. While current rhetoric supports participatory projects and doing communication better, the reality fits most often with earlier development models. And, at the same time, some older projects match current ideology in important elements. This smooth history will experience some fits and starts when it turns to the extended reviews of communication in agriculture and nutrition.

It is an unfinished history because, although the second-generation projects are well launched, we do not know how they will turn out. For the communication-as-complement projects, at least, the early work has gone well. However, their implementation over the long run and on a wide scale is yet to come. But if the history is unfinished, it can also still offer possibilities of success.

The history of communication for development, then, can be presented as a dialectic: problem, solution, problem, solution. As this is written, we are in a solution phase, with much exciting work ongoing. Surely there will be another problem phase to come; but for the moment, at least, despite the many problems of the past, there is reason for optimism.

The book elaborates this sketch of the field of communication for development, but its purpose is broader also. The historical view serves as an invaluable foundation, but the primary issue for many scholars and all practitioners has to be what can be built on that base. Can, in fact, communication for development have a more successful future than past? Under what conditions, for what objectives, and using what strategies will that success be realized?

The book proceeds through three parts. The next two chapters in Part One are conceptual and general. They extend these introductory comments. The first chapter expands the description of the roles communication has been asked to play in development programs. The second chapter, admitting that the greatest number of development projects fail, looks for explanations. It develops the hypotheses that guide the remainder of the book and prepares the ground for understanding proposed solutions.

Parts Two and Three review in substantial detail the place of communication in agriculture and in nutrition. They are the core of the book. At a straightforward level, they present a detailed history of attempts to affect agricultural practice and nutritional practice through information programs. However, in addition, they are an argument for a particular approach to communication for development. They do not assume that information is valuable; they start with an examination of evidence for the possibility of using information to affect particular agricultural or nutritional behaviors. The role of information in development cannot be understood without a fundamental understanding of particular agricultural or nutritional practices and their institutional and social context.

From the examination of the potential for using information, both the agriculture and nutrition reviews continue with a consideration of how conventional (nonmedia-based) programs have tried to provide such information. Comparison across programs stimulates the presentation of a list of problems with designing and implementing information programs in conventional ways. That in turn serves as a framework for analyzing the potential and realized contributions of media-based programs. At their best, it is argued, media-based programs do promise to resolve what has been the central problem of face-to-face education: organizing, maintaining, and paying for the necessary corps of field staff. Parts Two and Three are each reasonably complete and can be read independently of each other.

The concluding sections of Parts Two and Three present reviews and make specific recommendations. The book is thus an examination of evidence but ends by drawing conclusions in the form of implications for practice. Those implications are specific to agriculture and nutrition but generalize quite well to other areas of health and in a looser way to the application of communication to formal education.

The author has a personal history of involvement in communication for development research, and that involvement colors the interpretation of evidence and the conclusions drawn. If, therefore, readers examine the conclusions skeptically, all the better.

While the book has only one author, it is the fruit of a half-dozen specific research projects that involved the collaboration of a dozen other researchers, fifteen years of discussions with others interested in development communication, and specific reviews by those colleagues and others of parts of the manuscript.

Wilbur Schramm, John Mayo, and Emile McAnany have been teachers and collaborators and colleagues since 1968. I am not sure anymore which ideas are mine and which are theirs. Judith McDivitt worked with me on major sections of the manuscript, providing excellent advice that I sometimes accepted. Chapters 2 and 3 were first written when I was working on a project at Stanford University, reviewing communication policy for the U. S. Agency for International Development (Office of Education and Human Resources, Development Support Bureau). Collaborators on that project and on the background papers that were the sources for these two chapters included Ed Parker, who was co-principal investigator, and Ronny Adikharya, Eduardo Contreras-Budge, Dennis Foote, Doug Goldshmidt, Jeanne Moulton, Jeremiah O'Sullivan, Everett Rogers, Barbara Searle, and Doug Solomon, as well as Mayo and McAnany. The original version of the agriculture section was written under that sponsorship as well, with additional assistance from Sikandra Spain.

The nutrition section was written with support from the World Bank. A previous version was published by the United Nations Administrative Committee on Coordination, Subcommittee on Nutrition, as "Nutrition Policy Discussion Paper No. 1." Ideas for that manuscript and helpful comments on it came from Jere Behrman, Sidney Cantor, Jim Green, Marcia Griffiths, Jean-Pierre Habicht, Dean Jamison, Joanne Leslie, Gretel Pelto, Dave Radel, Richard Manoff, Tony Meyer, Tina Sanghvi, Bill Smith, Margaret Valdivia, Susan van der Vynct, and Marian Zeitlin. Alan Berg, Dave Gwatkin, and T. J. Ho were contract officers and offered substantial guidance. Doug Solomon coauthored a related study.

I am grateful to Cliff Block of USAID's Office of Education, both for his service as project officer on various funded research programs and in a much larger way for the opportunity to argue about communication for development. Tony Meyer of that office has so served more recently. Bill Smith and his colleagues at the Academy for Educational Development do impressive work in communication for development — work that is one explanation for the occasional optimism that is found here. It is not hard to trace Bill's influence on these pages.

Barbara Searle once promised to be my coauthor on this volume, but after contributing good ideas she thought better of it. It might have been done several years ago if she had stayed. Marsha Siefert was the editor for the book manuscript and provided invaluable advice on organization and on conceptual structure. I am grateful to her. Hillary Guenther, Maxine Beiderman, Susan DiNapoli, and Jane Whittendale prepared parts of the manuscript and Karen Wilkins developed the index.

This book belongs to my wife, Esther, and sons, Ben and Avram. I love them and am proud of them.

Development Communication

Part One

Communication and Development — An Overview

Chapter One

The Roles of Communication in Education/Information Projects

Communication technology has been used as a component in a variety of strategies for solving many different development problems. The subsequent sections describe these in some detail. First, however, some select examples serve to highlight the major functions of communication.

A functional analysis in the sociological tradition (Merton 1957) provides a useful framework for an examination of the place of communication in development. It lends two perspectives to our classification that are particularly to be valued. First, it tells us to look beyond manifest functions — the ostensible purpose of a program — to latent functions and dysfunctions — the effects, positive or negative, of a program's initiation, regardless of its sponsor's intentions. Second, it reminds us that the effects of a program are not restricted to the intended beneficiaries.

Many actors and institutions participate in a communication-for-development project. Each of these is affected by, and seeks various benefits from that participation. In understanding the character and social impact of a communication technology project, it is as important to describe the political benefits accruing to a sponsor as to describe the nutritional improvements among the target audiences. In the long run, outside observers may judge a program as a solution to the social problem to which it is directed. However, the specifics of how it works — the functions of communication for the sponsors, the internal project actors, and the intended beneficiaries — will tell us a great deal about whether and how that ultimate success is achieved.

COMMUNICATION AS LOW-COST LOUDSPEAKER

The extension of the expert voice at an acceptable cost is certainly the prime justification for the use of mass media in education/information projects. In formal education and also in agriculture or health, when local reception groups with a volunteer monitor make use of radio broadcasts, communication technology is used primarily to improve quality; in other sectors — for example, agriculture, family planning, and health projects — when rural target audiences are beyond the reach of the in-place extension network, communication technology is used to extend that network.

In Guatemala, agricultural politics and national budgets constrain the number of extension agents the Ministry of Agriculture can hire. The shortfall means that many subsistence farmers are not reached with information believed to be of value to them. With support from the U.S. Agency for International Development (USAID), an experimental program of daily agricultural radio broadcasts was started in 1973. Its purpose was to lead listening farmers to make substantial changes in farming practices in order to increase their crop yields. Replacing extension agents (or, more precisely, taking the place of needed but unavailable agents) with radio programs seemed to be a cheaper way of extending the voice of expertise, at least while the project remained in operation.

The project assumed (at least in its radio-only version — other versions complemented radio broadcasts with face-to-face communication) that there existed adoptable agricultural practices, using the resources available to the target farmers, that would significantly improve crop yield and profitability. It assumed that those practices could be adequately described over a series of radio broadcasts, and that the voice of the radio would be sufficiently authoritative that farmers would listen to it, believe it, and act on its recommendations. Even if the method were less successful than the face-to-face efforts of extension agents, its low cost might make it feasible as a substitute.

The project remains a good example of one use of communication as loudspeaker — extending the voice of expertise to areas where it would not otherwise be heard. As in this case, the loudspeaker is sometimes operating in the absence of alternative information distribution strategies.

A project in Nepal provides another example. Most Nepalese primary-school teachers are untrained, and the existing teacher education institutions are not able to train them within the foreseeable future. A radio-based distance education project is being implemented to extend the voice of the educator where there is no feasible alternative (Mayo et al. 1975; Graham and Paige 1981).

In other situations, there is an available local voice, but that voice is not considered adequate to the task at hand. In El Salvador, in the late 1960s, the government was determined to expand seventh- through ninth-grade enrollment. It was willing to construct some new classrooms and hire additional teachers, but recognized that the quality of instruction (none too high to start with) was sure to decline since the teachers who could be employed in the expanded system had training legally sufficient only for primary level. Instructional television was implemented to provide a master teacher in the classrooms of newly enrolled students and their newly upgraded teachers. By the mid-1970s enrollment in the seventh, eighth, and ninth grades had more than quadrupled; and the quality of instruction had been maintained or improved, at a cost per student lower than in the previous system (Mayo, Hornik, and McAnany 1976).

While communication is viewed primarily as a low-cost loudspeaker, it has played other roles in development. Some of these roles loom as large in our understanding of the function of communication technology as does the primary loudspeaker role. We turn to them now.

COMMUNICATION TECHNOLOGY AS INSTITUTIONAL CATALYST

In El Salvador, instructional television (ITV) was at the center of a substantial educational reform. ITV worked as a catalyst of that change in two ways. First, ITV's operating character demanded concomitant change in other components of the education system: curriculum specification and restructuring, reorganization of the school day, changes in classroom teaching styles, and development of teaching material like student workbooks and teacher's guides. All were needed to accommodate television. Second, ITV's political attractions mobilized sufficient momentum to overcome the inertia of the educational bureaucracy. Instructional television as the centerpiece of educational reform was chosen as a major campaign promise of the winning candidate for the presidency of El Salvador. As such, its political clout opened the way for many changes in the educational system. It is difficult to imagine that a textbook-based educational reform, regardless of its technical value, would have attracted similar support; consequently, one must doubt whether it would have catalyzed equal change in the system.

Many educational and information projects face similar traditional bureaucracies. Health ministries, with their emphasis on curative, hospital-bound services, are slow to shift funds to preventive or educational services. Introduction of communication technology-based programs, regardless of their effectiveness as compared to alternative strategies, may mobilize political forces outside of the ministry sufficient to achieve a substantial reallocation in priorities. Media-based projects have "star" quality and can attract support. At the same time, that star quality poses a risk, a point made in the following section.

COMMUNICATION AS POLITICAL LIGHTNING ROD

The proliferation in the developing world of "distance universities," following the British Open University model, is on the surface a respectable effort to meet a growing demand for higher education at a reasonable cost. At the same time, skeptics wonder whether those universities, at least in some cases, do not fulfill a political function rather more effectively than they do an educational one.

The population clamoring for access to university places is in most instances both a vociferous and politically potent force. After all, they are not subsistence peasants but the sons and daughters of the middle class. Governments ignore such demands at their peril. Distance universities provide a path to the satisfaction of those demands without straining construction budgets or available academic staff.

We know that the construction of effective courses within such institutions is an arduous task. Israel's open university (based on the British model) employs four to six professionals for one to two years in a typical course development effort (Melmed et al. 1982). However, the construction of courses may not be so demanding if effectiveness is not highly regarded. If a government can satisfy the political clamor by creating a distance program, it may not also recognize or respond to the additional demand that education be made effective. While outsiders may know that high dropout rates and poor learning are the consequences of badly constructed programs, the government may succeed in transferring the responsibility for such failure from the political system to the individual who had a chance but failed.

Communication programs can create the image of public action and give the appearance of political responsiveness; they earn political credit for their publicly identified progenitors. That they can serve such a short-term political function without necessarily serving a substantial development need is among the risks that advocates of communication technology must face. It is the underside of their ability to attract political support and gain institutional momentum. Technically appropriate strategies may be rejected in favor of politically appropriate media-based ones; this is a particular risk when it comes to what Wilbur Schramm (1977) called Big Media — for example, television and satellite transmissions. Political support attracted by technological charisma may not last the course when it comes down to providing the essential infrastructure to make the project work effectively.

COMMUNICATION AS ORGANIZER AND MAINTAINER

An innovation in an educational process can be excellently conceived and successful in enhancing learning in its early use, yet, over the long haul, fail to maintain that success. Teacher retraining as a route to improved classroom instruction may suffer this fate. The teacher may be shown valuable new techniques, but when he or she returns to the classroom, the working environment remains unchanged. Facing the frustration inherent in trial-and-error applications of new methods that precede their mastery, teachers may find it easy to slip back into customary practice. Contrast this pattern of innovation with that inherent in core use of radio or television for direct tutelage of students. In Nicaragua, the Radio Mathematics experiment (Friend et al. 1980) used thirty-minute, carefully developed radio broadcasts to teach mathematics to students in primary schools. Once the curriculum was completed, although modifiable, it represented a substantial obstacle against backsliding. It was there, every day, in the classroom, structuring mathematics instruction. It assured the necessary pace to move through the assigned curriculum. Teachers making use of prepared teacher's guides could extend or deepen instruction to the extent they were able, but the burden of maintaining the changed enviroment was not theirs. Once they decided to turn on the radio, the organization of the classroom day and the probability of maintaining the innovative educational process, not only during that year but in subsequent years, were enhanced. When used directly in an educational process, communication technology provides the backbone for organizing and maintaining change in a resistant environment.

The Tanzanian adult education authority used radio, in part, as the pivot of its nationwide campaigns in an analogous way (Hall and Dodds 1977). The ten- to twelve-week "Man Is Health" and other national campaigns organized discussion and decision groups (based on smaller preexisting political and adult education units) to listen and act after listening to weekly radio broadcasts about health (and other) problems and solutions. Clearly, national and local political forces were influential in the substantial success of these campaigns (evaluations reported the extraordinary figure of 700,000 latrines constructed). Nonetheless, the campaigns were organized around the radio broadcasts, which enabled the central planners to control the pace and structure of the activities.

In the United States, the Stanford Heart Disease Prevention Program illustrates another aspect of this organizing and maintaining function (Farquhar et al. 1975). This experimental program used mass media (as well as interpersonal communication for selected populations) to convince its target audience to change heart-disease-related behavior, including diet, exercise patterns, and smoking. However, short-term changes in behavior are not meaningful; new behavior patterns must be sustained in order to affect coronary health. In particular, changes in diet and exercise require daily decisions. The effects of educational programs that depend on a concentrated dose of information may fade as the treatment recedes in memory. Mass media campaigns, assuming they can lead to new behaviors in the first place (as in the Stanford program), can also reinforce the change with continuing reminders. That assumes, of course, an adequate budget to pay for repeated reinforcing messages.

Thus communication technology, used properly, may serve all three of these subfunctions, serving as the organizing structure for an educational process, maintaining an innovative process over an extended time, and reinforcing changes in behavior over time. Success in these roles is not inevitable; however, there has been some successful past experience in utilizing communication technology in these ways, and under the right conditions, such successes can be repeated.

COMMUNICATION AS EQUALIZER

Whether one considers the distribution of teachers or schooling resources, agricultural extension agents or health services, history provides an almost invariant lesson: The better off do better. The most experienced teachers, the better buildings, and what few textbooks are available go first to the urban schools, the schools of the relatively advantaged children. Agricultural extension agents reach the owners of larger farms but rarely the mass of subsistence farmers. Health services spread only slowly from urban and semiurban centers.

Unequal distribution of resources is inevitable as long as such resources are limited, and the ability of particular constituencies to make claims on those scarce resources is also unequal. One partial approach to that problem is to end the limits on resources so as to permit universal access. Communication media, in their capacity as loudspeaker, can provide such universal access.

In El Salvador, the instructional television system was the first school resource ever to be distributed equally across the seventh- through ninth-grade population. The fact that one school used the broadcast signal did not lessen the ability of other schools to make use of it, given that they all owned television receivers. In contrast, the fact that an urban school was able to attract an experienced teacher meant that a rural school could not.

Paradoxically, communication satellites, often viewed as the most high-technology, capital-intensive communication investment of all, can sometimes fulfill this equalizing function. In India, the Satellite Instructional Television Experiment (SITE) used the ATS-6 communication satellite to provide instruction to villages that would have been beyond the range of land-based broadcast distribution networks. Microwave and other conventional transmission networks usually spread outward slowly from the city. Satellite transmissions, in contrast, are distance independent. There is no need to first reach intermediate semiurban areas and then rural areas. The costs are largely the same whatever the location.

The equalizing potential is certainly here. Nonetheless two caveats must be entered. First, a nation must want to take advantage of this equalizing capability. Television signals may reach a school, but if no receiver has been purchased no benefit is possible. Similarly, satellites may make it less costly to reach distant regions, but again whether a nation is willing to or ought to commit the substantial absolute resources required for such a program is an open question.

Second, although communication technology promises an equalizing of access to opportunity, it does not necessarily promise an equalizing of benefits. Only some children arrived in El Salvador's seventh grade to take advantage of ITV (although many more than had taken advantage of traditional instruction). Only some people find that the agricultural advice available on radio broadcasts is actually helpful. Only some people have anyone to call when satellite technology brings telephone service to rural villages. While the design of both hardware and software of the communication system can affect equality of benefits, a substantial inequality will remain as a function of abilities and resources.

COMMUNICATION FOR IMPROVEMENT IN QUALITY

Early justification for instructional technology advocated spreading the voice of the master teacher and thus upgrading quality (whether in mathematics instruction or family-planning campaigns). It stressed duplicating the best of face-to-face instruction. There is another way to examine the quality issue, however. If constrained to duplicate face-to-face instruction, using media merely as loudspeaker, some decline in quality is inevitable. However, if one takes advantage of the special qualities of a variety of media, maximizing the potential of each, one may develop a different instructional process, equal to or better than high-quality face-to-face instruction.

A good illustration of such maximizing is the program design for the Radio Mathematics project. The group providing technical assistance brought ten years of experience in constructing mathematics curricula for computer-assisted instruction to the creation of the radio-based curriculum. The project staff spent one year in developing each grade's programming: designing curriculum, producing programs with a complex and artful understanding of how mathematics is learned, and gathering extensive feedback from classroom observation and testing. Knowing that each program was to be used and reused, the directors could justify a heavy investment in software development. Programs were produced or, more precisely, new curricula were developed that no master teacher was likely to duplicate.

The recent resurgence in distance education following the model of the British Open University illustrates the same issue (Perraton 1982). While correspondence education, including television or other media, has had a long history, it often has been one of high dropout rates and dreary instruction. The contrasting success of the British effort and of similar ones elsewhere, including Everyman's University in Israel, has been due in no small way to the care with which the instructional package was developed. As with Radio Mathematics, each course combined radio and television broadcasts with textbooks, exercises, and some face-to-face review. Rather than duplicating the traditional educational process, these institutions struck out on their own, taking maximum advantage of all the channels of communication at their disposal.

COMMUNICATION TECHNOLOGY AS ACCELERATOR OF INTERACTION

In Alaska, small rural villages had only a health aide, a member of the community who was given six weeks of training, to provide ordinary health care (Hudson and Parker 1973). To support the limited skills and experience of those aides, the health system introduced two-way radios (eventually using a satellite to improve transmission quality) that provided daily contact with physicians at regional hospitals. While some slower form of communication might have been possible (mail planes irregularly arrived at the villages and might have taken messages), clearly the character of the resulting health system would have been very different.

Rural people depend on communication with more populated areas for many aspects of their lives. Agricultural seed and fertilizer may come from outside, and cash crops are sold outside; consumer goods may be manufactured elsewhere; schools and health posts are supplied and supervised, if at all, by central offices; laborers may need to locate plantation work at a distance. All of these relations with distant centers require communication. Such interaction can be accelerated substantially by communication technology and, as in the Alaska example, make a qualitative difference in the character of some of those interactions. We do not know, however, the implications of this acceleration. We do not know which relations would be largely unaffected, which would work to the advantage of rural participants, and which to their disadvantage.

COMMUNICATION AS LEGITIMATOR/MOTIVATOR

Because something is broadcast over the mass media, it must be important; conversely, if something is important, it will surely be broadcast over the media. Some sophisticated observers think they are inured to what sociologists Paul Lazarsfeld and Robert Merton (1948) called the "status conferral" function of mass media. It is an arguable point. Nonetheless, we suspect that for most people in the world, mass media retain this special credibility. Thus social advertisers use radio to sell "Superlimonada," a rehydration formula, to combat infant diarrhea (Cooke and Romweber 1977). And while radio serves as a loudspeaker that provides access to large audiences, the fact that the messages are on the radio gives them credibility for each listener. In a curiously circular logic, advertisers buy audience-reach and because they bought reach, they have bought credibility.

The credibility lent by access to mass media may extend elsewhere. The constant broadcasting of a national language, anthems, and other national symbols both teaches that language and those symbols and legitimizes them. A family-planning radio campaign may be no more effective per dollar investment in reaching audiences than alternative channels, but its extra credibility may affect adoption. Regular television broadcasts may motivate attendance at agricultural discussion groups, even if the content could equally well have been presented locally.

Some might argue that an additional legitimizing function of the mass media is the most profound of all. Sensitization of policy-making elites, and their consequent involvement in policy change in such areas as population and nutrition, may affect the success of development programs more than direct interactions with target audiences can. Mass media presentation may legitimate a particular problem justifying national attention and thereby increase access for interested groups to the policy-making process.

COMMUNICATION FOR FEEDFORWARD

It has been customary to focus on the role of communication technology either in solving problems of message distribution to mass audiences or in accelerating interaction between individuals. However, an additional role involves the use of communication technology to magnify the ability of individuals in a population to speak to the central institutions that affect them.

In its simplest form this involves the publication of letters to the editors of mass circulation newspapers focusing attention on one problem or another. In Senegal's "Radio Dissou" program, the letters-to-the-editor notion was transferred to a broadcast medium (Cassirer 1977). Seventy percent of the broadcast materials were expressions of viewpoints, complaints, and questions from rural audiences. The rest were responses by government agencies to those comments or the provision of useful information. It was reported that substantial modifications of government policy were the result of the large-scale peasant use of this feedforward channel.

The agriculture sector is one in which the need for feedforward is most acute. Agricultural research agencies, it is argued, are often unresponsive to the needs of subsistence farmers, in part because they have no regular means of hearing from those farmers through influential channels. If correct, the argument calls for a *feedforward channel* that both communicates the changing character of those needs and enters the agricultural research policy institutions in an influential way (McDermott 1971).

Obviously, in both the realized Senegal case and in the hypothetical agricultural case, the success of the feedforward channel in influencing policy will depend on how open the policy-making apparatus is to such information. In Senegal, President Senghor overruled the attempt of the directors of criticized government services to have Radio Dissou silenced. In many countries the agricultural feedforward channel will never be created, will be quashed, or will be ineffectual unless substantial political interests guarantee its role.

COMMUNICATION AS MAGNIFIER
OF DEPENDENCY/INTEGRATION

Communication reinforces the links between participants. The statement is obvious; what is not so obvious is the interpretation, or the desirability, of that result. As we have seen, improved communication for agricultural marketing has the potential for both benefits *and* exploitation. Similarly, what to a government broadcast authority is the sharing of a national language and symbols to foster nation building, is to its critics the systematic derogation of minority cultures. In each case the optimistic view (or the view of those with control over the technology) is that of beneficial integration; for those to be integrated, fearing exacerbation of already-existing unequal status, the introduction of specific communication technology programs may suggest increased dependency.

That point can be made at a more general level also. Sophisticated communication technology, it has been argued, leaves its users at the mercy of those who control that technology. At the national level that may mean that central institutions increase their dominance of national information networks. An illustration — at the risk of oversimplification — may make the point. When many itinerant entertainers and news carriers are replaced by a national radio station, multiple and most likely diverse sources of information are replaced by more efficient, more entertaining, and potentially more accurate, but often more homogeneous government-controlled information sources.

The national dependence argument has its international parallel. Small countries like El Salvador must import all of their technology, from transmitters and receivers to videotape for their ITV systems. Often only equipment from a single supplier is compatible with in-place systems. A shift in political climate can leave users stranded and faced with unexpected costs, or it can force them to comply with what they consider interference in their own policies. This vulnerability is extreme when countries are faced with the huge capital costs of purchasing and launching a satellite. A nation that, for example, leases time on a foreign-controlled satellite for its domestic communications network may perceive itself as risking substantial reduction in national autonomy during times of conflict. This fear of dependency has been voiced in the debates in developing countries over the appropriateness of satellites.

COMMUNICATION PROGRAMS FOR CREATING AND SUPPLYING DEMAND

Some sectors face problems of supplying demand, others those of creating demand. The demands for formal education, agricultural information, curative health services, and sometimes contraceptives, for example, are well established and are often greater than government agencies can satisfy; the task is to increase the supply of services or information. As an illustration, broadcast instruction may permit expansion of the school system through larger classes and the employment of less well-trained and less well-paid teachers while maintaining quality. Radio farm forums extend the distribution of agricultural information.

Other sectors are more concerned with problems of creating demand. Non-formal education programs may need to generate audience interest for literacy, health, and nutrition courses. The lack of demand for such services, of course, raises questions about how useful they are. However, the perceived value of such services sometimes may be less than the "objective" value that justifies attempts to generate new demand. Demand-creating projects are particularly appropriate when new resources are available.

The implications for project formulation of this demand-supply distinction are important. If the problem is defined as one of supply, investments go first to efficient distribution systems, developing cheaper ways of making education available or of increasing public knowledge about services. Demand problems call first for investment in motivation and in mechanisms (like group meetings and multiple channels) that ease and reinforce participation.

It is possible to overplay the distinction, however, A project that is organized to supply a service may find that preexisting demand is limited to a narrow stratum, and that the people most in need of the service (whether it be education, agricultural information, or contraceptive devices) do not respond to simple increased availability. If such projects are to achieve significant social change, they must see themselves, before very long, as demand-creating projects also.

There are, in sum, a wide range of roles that communication technology has been asked to play, or does play regardless of whether or not it was meant to do so. We have illustrated each of those roles with specific projects and have located the roles within relevant contexts. While there have been questioning comments here and there, by and large this section has described potential functions; it has not considered the conditions under which those functions have been realized. In fact, most attempts to use communication to achieve development outcomes have fared poorly. In the next chapter, we examine alternative explanations for why success has been rare.

Chapter Two

Why Communication for Development So Rarely Succeeds

There are, in the developing world, several thousand educational programs now operating that use communication technology to reach their objectives. These programs employ mass media, two-way communication technology, and miscellaneous audiovisual devices in formal education, adult education, information campaigns, development administration, and all manner of community development programs. Given the available data about audiences reached, practices changed, benefits achieved, and long-term institutional survival, we can assume that most of them fail; they have not reached even a small part of their apparent goals. It is our purpose to understand these failures and the few successes and, insofar as we can, locate circumstances that promise success.

Following Suchman (1967), we first divide the explanations for failure into two broad categories: theory failures (resulting from an incorrect assumption that a particular development problem is amenable to a communication-based solution) and program failures (resulting from an inadequately designed or implemented project). We also add a third category: political failures. Each type of failure will be introduced and discussed at a general level; in Parts Two and Three, detailed support for these propositions will be offered in relation to particular substantive goals.

THEORY FAILURES

Projects based on communication technology traffic in information. They throw words — ways of understanding, behaving, and organizing — at development problems, problems that are substantially and contrarily defined as a lack of resources: low agricultural productivity, poor health or nutritional status, or unequal shares of society's goods.

To argue that information provision alone can resolve development problems is to assume that available resources are being inefficiently used. It is to argue that substantially more benefit can be derived from what is already in place, if only individuals or groups knew better how to organize the use of those resources: additional agricultural products can result from improved farming practices without the introduction of expensive fertilizers; infants' nutritional status can be improved with better feeding and health practices, although no new food is available to the family and no new medical facilities are available in the community. In both of these examples, the assumption is that current behavior is irrational — it is not producing the maximum benefit from the available resources. People do not know, so they do not act optimally. This assumption of human deficit — of individual ignorance as to how to make the best use of the available resources — although rarely explicit, was central to much communication for development practice.

Yet most scholars who have looked closely at agricultural or nutritional practices, for example, claim that the assumption of irrationality is inappropriate. It is often inappropriate in the economic sense: it is common to find, for example, that small farmers are highly efficient users of available resources (Schultz 1964). It is also often inappropriate in the cultural sense: the benefits accrued are not limited to economic returns. For example, current weaning practices may reinforce valued social ties, even if they fail to maximize other valued goals. Indeed, if current practice fits into its economic and cultural milieu, then development strategies that depend entirely on providing information have little potential for success.

This strong statement may explain why many projects fail; let us therefore look for ways around it. If communication-based projects are essentially providers of information, under what circumstances do they have a positive developmental role? Four perspectives offer promise. The first two point to situations where current behavior is not optimum and suggest that communication can accelerate the process of adaptation to a changed environment.

The first perspective suggests that there are, in fact, important situations where current behavior is tightly linked neither to a culture nor to its economy. A rapidly changing environment can make a previously well adapted behavior no longer optimum. A growing population means that available land must be divided into parcels too small for subsistence; or it may force some people to become laborers on plantations or to migrate to cities. Changes in international commodity prices or in distribution possibilities affect which crops are sown and thus alter food prices. National upheavals — revolutions, wars, or natural disasters — dictate rapid changes in the social organization of communities. In each of these circumstances older practices no longer fit, and people may be open to newer ones that fit better with the changing environment. Provision of information under such ripe circumstances may find fertile ground for influencing the direction of change.

A second way around the assumption that current behavior is, in fact, well adapted, is to use communication in a broader program that is introducing new resources. The availability of new resources by itself implies a change in the environment that has reinforced existing behavior. Thus new programs of low-cost agricultural credit mean that farmers are making decisions according to new criteria and may value information about how to maximize benefits under these previously unknown conditions. Information is also of value when a new product or technology, whether it be a new soy milk blend or corn hybrid, becomes available. Informing people about both the nature and availability of a new product and the specifics of its use are potential roles.

However, if the comparative advantage of the new products or technology is very large, the need for information may be satisfied through the natural information-sharing process and no formal information campaign may be required. Thus the value of information campaigns is bounded on the one hand by an unchanging environment that does not reward new behaviors, and on the other by an environment changed by the availability of new resources whose applicability is so clear as to require no complementary information campaign.

A third way of addressing the assumption that current practices fit the environment is to argue that not all programs of information and education are means to a subsequent development end; they can be an end in themselves. Becoming politically informed or educated in basic skills is a social good, and not merely because either leads to better agricultural or nutritional practice and then higher income. This perspective assumes that education programs are in themselves new resources and their availability represents a change in the environment. People will consume the programs because the programs have intrinsic value. Their acceptance is not conditioned by the value of what is learned for other purposes.

This view of education as a social good, and thus not troubled by the irrationality problem, is, of course, not universally shared. Human capital theorists (cf. Schultz 1964; Welch 1970; Jamison and Lau 1982; Behrman and Wolfe 1984) assume that better-skilled people will use available resources more efficiently, and that education is to be valued precisely because it helps individuals rationalize their use of resources. Others argue that economic opportunity is related to educational attainment, especially when pressures on the land increase. Only if education is linked to economic advantage will it be sought. Both alternative views suggest that investments in educational programs, no less than in more obviously practice-related information programs, will pay off only if they are related to environmental disequilibria that enhance their value.

The fourth approach to the "practice fits" obstacle is to stress the organizational value of communication as opposed to its informative value. Some would argue that information from outside a community will not affect that community unless it starts a process of autonomous development. From this perspective the value of communication programs is not in the specific practices they advocate, but in the local organization and longer-term political activism they generate. Associated with the terms "consciousness-raising" and "community development" (each from rather different political traditions), this approach accepts the notion that information delivered to, and for the use of, the individual peasant is of little value. Failure to develop is not the result of individual incapacity. Rather, even though individuals, on the average, may maximize their own use of resources, communities do not. There is residual power in effective organization of the community. From the community development perspective, that means improvements in the standard of living can be achieved by adopting innovations (such as roads or a water supply) that are beyond the resources of the individual but within those of the organized community. From the consciousness-raising perspective, this means that communities can make effective demands on outside political authority for a more equitable share of national resources.

Communication programs that are designed to mobilize community organization are thus held to be free from the assumption of individual deficits in their efforts to accelerate development. They do assume a parallel "community deficit," that community failure to develop is not a reflection of true resource constraints or true lack of power, but is, at least in part, due to a failure to make use of resources and power that are potentially available. And further, it is assumed that outside stimulation of local organization is an effective means of initiating the realization of that potential.

We then have four broad classes of potential uses of communication: in the context of rapid environmental change, as a component of a program introducing new resources, as an end in itself, and for purposes of community organization for development. Each recognizes that information alone is rarely a satisfactory solution to resource-based development problems. Development programs that do not use communication in one of these ways, no matter how well designed those programs are in a technical sense, have little promise of success. They fail because their theory of the role of communication in development is inadequate.

However, even programs that do make more reasonable assumptions about communication's role may not find the going easy. We turn now to our second broad category of explanation for failure: program failures due to an inadequately designed or implemented project.

PROGRAM FAILURES

Effective projects using communication technology are technology projects only to the naive observer. Two projects may make identical hardware purchases, and with the same intention, but produce entirely different results. What counts is what is done with the hardware. While this is commonplace wisdom to those who are experienced in media-based instructional projects, it is not always shared by the enthusiasts who are responsible for the creation of the many projects that appear each year around the world. Excited by the extraordinary reach of a medium, they may not invest sufficiently beyond the hardware to have any hope of success. Nonhardware considerations include macro- and microinstructional design, obtaining information from the field, administrative location of communication projects, and internal-to-the-project staffing and organizational decisions.

Macroinstructional Design

In some schemes, providing an item of information will have its intended effect on some proportion of an intended audience even if it is transmitted over a single channel only once. "You have the job — start Monday." "No credit available." However, such straightforward circumstances are rare, or so much of the codified experience suggests (cf. Schramm 1977; Jamison and McAnany 1978; Rogers 1983). Projects that depend on a single medium to reach their audiences may find that some part of the audience is inaccessible or does not entirely understand, or if it does understand does not use the medium as a stimulus for practice change. Projects that use multiple channels have a higher probability of success, both because different channels serve different needs and because redundancy is of intrinsic value. Support for these propositions comes from diffusion theory and instructional design theory.

Scholars of the diffusion of innovation have argued persuasively that the adoption of new behaviors should be viewed as a multistage process. The particular sequence of such stages varies (Rogers, for example, opts for knowledge, persuasion, decision, and confirmation) but the proposed sequence is not important. What matters is the perception of innovation as a process, with the adopter and his or her community using information from outside to satisfy different needs at different stages in the process.

If the needs for information vary with the adoption stage, then the communication channel most appropriate for delivering that information may vary also. For example, a common diffusion model suggests that in the knowledge stage, as individuals become aware of an innovation, they rely on mass media; as individuals move toward a decision, they tend to rely on personal sources. However, one need have no faith in this particular formulation to accept the more general premise.

Indeed, it will be useful to take a broader view than is typical in diffusion research. Needs to be served by an information system can be differentiated on intra- and interindividual and intertopic dimensions. Diffusion theorists emphasize the changing cognitive and psychological context as the innovator moves toward adoption; they focus on intraindividual changes. A channel that can effectively provide information about what is available needs to be replaced by a channel that can assure the individual of community support for change or one that can establish the legitimacy of the innovation for the local context. A channel that effectively supplies ideas may need to be replaced by a channel that gives the innovator the opportunity to clarify doubts, or that promises personal interaction if things go wrong.

Another dimension of needs to be considered addresses inter- rather than intraindividual variation. All channels of communication do not reach all members of the audience equally well, whether for reasons of physical access or because of differences in learned skills. Agricultural extension agents reach some farmers but not others; radio ownership is by no means universal in the rural areas of developing countries. Even when a medium physically reaches an individual, it may not serve as an effective communication channel. Literacy in a medium varies whether that involves reading pamphlets, understanding radio messages, or talking to socially distant extension agents.

A final dimension of needs looks not within or across individuals but across content areas. Some topics seem to require more or less visual support of verbal messages, or other channel capacities related to the way they are most easily presented. Sometimes a mechanism for storing information locally is required; sometimes it is essential for individuals to control the pace of their exposure to information; at other times externally paced exposure is to be valued. While many channels are feasible for satisfying each of these needs, some channels are likely to be more effective than others.

The argument for multiple channel systems has yet another support. One of the communication stategies that has proved most effective in achieving development goals is that of *mobilization*. All available media concentrate national attention on a particular problem. In Tanzania (Hall and Dodds 1977), China (Chu 1977), and Cuba (Fagen 1969), multiple channels (broadcast and print mass media, local groups, schools, and political institutions) concentrate massive national efforts on selected social goals — whether improved health practices, the elimination of landlords, or the promotion of literacy. The strength of multiple channels in these instances is not in their differentiation of roles but in their redundancy. The sense of national mobilization is communicated by the use of multiple channels per se, regardless of the content assigned to each medium.

The general argument for multiple-channel communication systems is rather easier to make than is the definition of just what communication needs a program has and what channels are likely to serve these needs most effectively. We hold no brief for a very tight match between needs and channels. Obviously the particular sectorial, financial, and institutional constraints under which a project operates will restrain its options. Also it is one thing to argue for multiple channels; no doubt more is better. It is quite another to administer and pay for them, which suggests more may not be optimum. In any case, comments about the specifics of this matter must be left to the chapters that address particular sectorial applications. However, one example may illustrate the argument.

An in-service teacher-training program may require (1) the transmission of information, (2) a chance to review material at one's own pace, (3) the chance to practice newly learned techniques and obtain constructive feedback, (4) motivation to maintain attention over the long haul, (5) an opportunity to clarify doubts, (6) a sense of membership in a community going through a common program, (7) an outside stimulus to maintain the pace of learning.

Daily radio broadcasts might be effective for tasks 1, 4, 5, and 7; a programmed text might serve 1 and 2; observation by supervisors or organized assistance of school principals of in-class teaching would help tasks 3 and 5; and brief periods of resident instruction might meet the need for 2, 3, 4, 5, and 6. Choosing such a combination of redundant and complementary channels matched to the information needs of a particular program addresses the macroinstructional design issue. However, choosing a useful configuration of channels is valuable only if it is followed by the effective use of the channels that are chosen.

Microinstructional Design

It is unlikely that one could find a planning document for a media-based educational project that states that there is no need to prepare good content materials once one has invested in the hardware. In fact, however, that has been the consequence of the pattern of staffing and budgeting that many projects have followed. As an extreme example, in Samoa, a single teleteacher was responsible for between 10 and 20 televised grade school programs per week, in addition to writing classroom materials! As Schramm suggests (1973, 48), such "ITV programs are not going to win any prizes." However, that is an early example; and neither in Samoa currently nor, to our knowledge, in most other programs are such unreasonable demands made on producers. If, however, programs have moved toward greater emphasis on quality in content, that has turned out to have two quite distinct meanings.

The first, and perhaps more common, approach emphasizes aesthetic quality. It encompasses both technical accomplishments (clarity of sound reproduction, smoothness of editing) and creative accomplishment (variety of settings, quality of acting, and intrinsic entertainment value). The model is commercial programming, and the standards those of the production fraternity. While certainly there is nothing wrong with achievement of aesthetic quality, it is not what we emphasize when we speak of quality. And unfortunately the emphasis on aesthetic quality has led more than one program astray.

When we speak of quality in instructional design, we refer to pedagogical quality: logical structure to the curriculum, effective building on the existing experiences of the audience, and devices to make sure that audiences are actively involved in mental processing. The quality of educational materials is not measured by the applause of colleagues and critics but by their effectiveness. Pedagogical quality is the result not merely of investment in studio facilities and talented producers but in the support of a linked system of audience analysis, curriculum design, program production, pretesting, field utilization, and feedback. In contrast to the Samoan example, the Radio Mathematics project in Nicaragua produced but five programs per week with a staff of fourteen professionals. A substantial proportion of staff time was spent maintaining links with the classroom audience, and all but two members of the staff (one Nicaraguan, one expatriate) were educators rather than broadcasters (Friend et al. 1980). It is true that the capital costs of curriculum development were high, and thus the effort is perhaps not directly replicable in many other circumstances. Nonetheless, the basic commitment to quality in instructional design is worth emulating.

Obtaining Information from the Field

Communication projects make assumptions about what is true in the environment of their intended beneficiaries, an environment that may be at a substantial geographic and cultural distance from the projects' sponsors and staff. Because of that distance, intrinsic to the use of communication technology, those assumptions will rarely serve as the basis for a successful project. The need for the confirmation of assumptions through the gathering of data is considerable both at the time a project is being planned, and at the time it is being implemented. The natural feedback cues that constrain face-to-face communication must be replaced with explicit data-gathering mechanisms in systems that rely on communication technology.

At the planning phase, a recommendation that a particular nutrition-related practice be adopted assumes that the new practice will indeed be more advantageous than the old one. A program to deliver market price information over the radio assumes that current knowledge is inadequate and farmers can act on new information. Both assumptions demand evidence.

At the time of implementation, a message strategy that assumes that economic motivations for a particular nutritional practice are paramount may be misguided if the current behavior is largely supported by important social bonds. Similarly, market price broadcasts may be useless if the pricing unit is one the audience is unfamiliar with or if the information is not available when they have surpluses.

Projects that operate at a distance, as communication projects do, are in constant need of information for planning and for adjusting operations. They need to know what is going well and what is not. They need both efficient data-gathering mechanisms and, no less, time and flexibility within their operational structures to define the information that can be used to take full advantage of the information that is gathered.

Administrative Locations of Communication Projects

Organizers of communication for development usually choose one of three administrative locations for their projects. The predominant mode is to locate communication projects within the substantive ministry concerned. Formal education projects like the El Salvador ITV project or the Korean Educational Development Institute are undertaken by ministries of education, for example, with secondary roles played by public or private communication institutions that help with transmission.

A second strategy is to locate projects within the communication ministry (posts and telegraphs, telecommunication, or whatever its title) or national radio or TV service. This is always the strategy if rural telephone service is the object, but it also may be chosen for projects with substantive goals. These offices, it is believed, will be able to share scarce skills broadly and service the needs of a number of institutions. Indonesia and Liberia, for example, have created development communication agencies to serve different substantive agencies. Many national broadcasting operations, particularly those influenced by the British model, have rural or development broadcasting units. Radio Gambia, for example, coordinates the production of programs for agriculture, health, schools, and other governmental agencies.

A third strategy is to create a hybrid agency by drawing on two or more institutions. These include agencies created for a specific project (Colombia's INRAVISION for its primary ITV project and Guatemala's National Out-of-School Education Board are examples) and agencies of a broader gauge (integrated rural development projects like Plan Puebla in Mexico) in which a communication component will play a secondary role.

Realistically, which strategy is chosen will depend on the overall character of the project and, particularly, its political genesis and support. In that context, experience from elsewhere may be irrelevant. However, when there is some flexibility in the decision, the arguments for the first mode seem to be the strongest. Placing communication within the substantive agency concerned recognizes that communication must complement a broader intervention. It serves to accelerate change, not instigate it. Success of a communication intervention will depend on joint action with field agents or the timely distribution of resources.

Projects organized outside the agency that employs the agents or owns the resources cannot count on their long-term availability, no matter how sincere the promises of cooperation at the outset. The centrifugal pull of institutional jealousies, rooted in competition for scarce resources, is going to be too great. In general, projects cannot succeed if they are not guaranteed the long-term support of the substantive agency, and they are not likely to achieve that support outside of that authority. The argument closely reflects our belief that communication investments must respect the existing development context, no matter how tempting it is ignore it and rely on the power of the technology. Nonetheless, we do recognize two powerful counterarguments. One is that a substantive authority is not easily galvanized; and while communication projects can be impressive catalysts to change, they may be insufficient to move an entrenched bureaucracy. The second is that projects organized within single agencies make rational telecommunication hardware planning difficult.

Sensible telecommunication hardware investment for a single substantive project will be very different from that for a large number of projects aggregated across agencies and over time. A radio production studio and some air time on a national radio network may make sense for an agricultural information project. No such project can justify a widespread rural telephone network. A single substantive project that proposed such an investment (or similarly costly ones involving satellites or the use of television in rural areas) would not even be considered. Yet if an existing system could be used for its marginal or average cost, different sets of considerations would come into play and such projects might be funded.

However, if projects remain under the independent control of substantive authorities, how is demand to be aggregated so as to produce a telecommunication system that is rationalized for all uses? The dilemma is real and it is not solved by letting things take their course. Under natural forces, the pattern of tele-communication investment is likely to reflect commercial — particularly urban — interests, leaving rural development concerns in second or third place. Systems inappropriate for development communication uses may be the result.

In the abstract, a hybrid agency with representatives of all communication-using institutions advising the telecommunications ministry would be ideal. However, it is not clear how this will provide funding for development telecommunication, unless the advice is accompanied by binding commitments for budget subventions. In most nations, telecommunication agencies are expected to pay their own way; a change in that policy will require some new source of funds and new political commitments.

Staffing and Organizational Decisions
Internal to the Project

This is a final catch-all category. It is the tautological refuge of the planner whose parting words to those charged with implementing a project are: "Do everything else right and the project will work, but if it didn't work you didn't do everything else right." Everything else includes hiring well-trained, competent, and committed staff, locating a charismatic central figure, establishing working conditions and supervisory relations that permit people to reach their potential, and developing effective links between the central office and the field staff. Such circumstances are obviously ideal; the question of interest is how to realize them. Why is it that some projects employ staff who do wonders despite difficult conditions, and others, with every chance of success, flounder because of internal failures?

Three types of answers are worth considering. The first, and least helpful, credits individual judgment and luck. A given program happened to find a talented leader who chose subordinates intelligently, and together they made it work. There are real individual differences in competence, and often they are difficult to detect until people are at work on the job. By happenstance, some projects have better staffs than others. How often this is a primary explanation, we do not know. However, if it is the primary explanation, short of noble pronouncements about the need for the careful selection of staff, there is little to be said that is both general and helpful.

The second type of answer looks to the character of communication technology projects per se. They have both advantages and disadvantages in the competition for talented staff and in the creation of effective organization. On the advantage side, any project that uses mass media retains a special glamor and promise of public notice and that is often an advantage in recruiting talented staff. Also, since the tasks undertaken by a media production unit, for example, have no parallel in traditional government bureaucracies, such units have a relatively free hand in developing an appropriate organizational structure. On the disadvantage side, it is often the case that enthusiastic young recruits do not fit well in the traditional bureaucracy that surrounds them and is jealous of their special status. Also, both the demands of the production process, and the media tradition that rewards aesthetic rather then pedagogical success, mitigate against maintaining close links with audiences of field staffs. The public visibility of media projects may mean that their staff is held more accountable than the staff of other projects, which may exaggerate the search for scapegoats at times of failure. That does not make for easy working relationships.

The special characteristics of communication technology projects thus define the second answer. The third answer suggests that failures of personnel and organization may not be technical program failures at all. The project leaders' lack of qualifications for their tasks, governmental red tape that disallows the paying of appropriate salaries, and a budget insufficient to pay for vehicles and field expenses may appear to be "mere" technical failures. After all, we know about the shortage of qualified personnel, the rigidity of government bureaucracies, and the shortfall of budgets. Yet in each of those cases, we are seeing the consequences of allocation decisions that are the result of a political process. If there is no money for a field operation, although it seems essential for success, if a project leader evidences more political loyalty than management competence, we are seeing not technical failures but failures of political will. The public appearance of taking action that is achieved easily by communication technology projects may satisfy the interests of project sponsors. The additional political commitments required to win adequate budget allocations and to survive bureaucratic infighting, commitments that produce successful development outcomes, may not be forthcoming.

This last reason for failure leads us to a final category of explanation. It is both independent of, but often associated with, theoretical and technical program failures.

THE POLITICAL EXPLANATION OF FAILURE

Communication technology projects, as with most development projects, will rarely succeed without prior commitment to change in the sector by substantial political forces. In earlier, more naive times, communication enthusiasts had hoped that their awesome technologies might somehow circumvent current political interests. By changing the organization and speed of information distribution, they argued, the distribution of power and society's goods could also be changed.

However, four decades of experience have taught us that the technologies, awesome as they may be, are under the control of those interests. The information that is to be transmitted and the feedback that will be heard are defined by those who control the hardware.

Mathematics education can be improved through the use of radio. But it will not be unless a real commitment to change is reflected in salaries adequate to attract and retain high-quality production personnel, time and facilities to produce good programs, encouragement and training for teachers, and availability of sufficient resources to implement and maintain the project broadly.

Agricultural radio, which informs farmers of innovative ways to plant their crops, will have little impact if the fertilizer the farmers need is unavailable or too expensive, if the market system cannot absorb the surplus, or if the costs of credit, the insecurity of land tenancy, and the vagaries of weather make the innovation too risky.

Such failures perhaps ought not be viewed as failures at all; rather, they are accurate reflections of current political interests. In the creation of any project, there are always competing interests both at the level of commitment to the expressed goals of a project and at the level of particular emphases within a project. This may mean that the needs of subsistence farmers fail to guide what agricultural researchers do because others have first call on research institutions. Broadcast primary school instruction may be stymied if other priorities like university education or teacher salaries have first call on available resources. The addition of an interactive communication capacity to a health project will not produce change if most variation in the success of health treatment is not due to ignorant health aides but to an unwillingness to provide medicines or an inability to provide transportation to a hospital.

The list can go on, but the implication is clear. At the risk of repetition: project failure often is not merely a technical failure or a failure of management; rather, technical and management failings may be symptoms of the distribution of power in a society. Communication interventions should be undertaken when concrete evidence of commitment to change in the sector is present. This would take the form of an adequate budget, talented and politically central managers, and, more broadly, promising field conditions. Because communication projects are glamorous, they easily attract superficial political support. It is the more fundamental support, which is essential when the communication intervention complements concomitant and politically difficult change in other areas, that is harder to come by.

These then are the hypotheses that guide our presentation. We think we understand some development contexts that offer ripe circumstances for the use of communication technology. We think we understand the program design strategies that enhance the probability of success. In Parts Two and Three, we begin to look at the evidence for our propositions.

We have chosen to focus on just two sectors: agriculture and nutrition. This concentration occurs although the educational and informational use of communication technology is important in other sectors (for example, formal schooling, nonformal education, health, and population) and potentially significant in additional ones (for examples, development administration, and community development). Nonetheless, most of the central arguments can be illustrated clearly with reference to these two sectors, supplemented by examples drawn from other applications. And concentrating our attention on just two sectors permits a more thoroughgoing review than would otherwise be possible.

Part Two focuses on agriculture and Part Three on nutrition. In each case we begin with an examination of arguments and evidence that information investments are important in the sector. We want to know whether and when it makes theoretical sense to throw information at problems. Next we present descriptions of conventional education/information programs in each sector. We look for evidence that they are effective and also analyze the types of problems such programs typically face. Finally, and at some length, we examine strategies that make use of communication technology — again looking at evidence of effectiveness as well as typical difficulties.

Part Two

Communication and Agriculture

Chapter Three

The Roles of
Information in Agriculture

Agriculture remains the primary source of employment for the majority of the world's population. Some 61 percent of the population of the developing world is employed in agriculture and 18 percent of its gross domestic product is derived from the land (World Bank 1979). Despite increased urbanization and growth of the industrial and service sectors, more people each year are working in the agricultural sector (and of course more people are dependent on agricultural products) than in the previous year. The growth in the productive capacity of the agricultural sector is crucial to the survival and development of most less-developed countries (LDCs).

In most areas of the developing world, the quantity of land available to agriculture is fixed or declining. The intrinsic quality of land apparently accounts for little of the interregional and intercountry difference in productivity (Schultz 1964). A surplus of labor is often available; but an expanded labor force, given a fixed land supply, is unlikely to yield a substantial increase in product relative to its cost. Thus neither land nor labor increases are likely to boost agricultural product. Most observers then turn to technological improvement as the most promising path to agricultural growth (Schultz 1964; Hayami and Ruttan 1971).

Changes in material inputs, complementary farming techniques, storage technology, and research, supply, and marketing institutions are all part of the technological transformation. The effective integration of these factors, it is argued, is tied closely to adequate information flows. In the words of Hayami and Ruttan:

A continuous stream of new technical knowledge and a flow of industrial inputs in which the new knowledge is embodied represents a necessary condition for modern agricultural development. This stream of inputs must be complemented by investments in general education and in production education for farmers and by efforts to transform institutions to be consistent with the new growth potentials.... The critical element in this process is an effective system of market and non-market information linkage among farmers, public research institutions, private agricultural supply firms, and the markets for products (1971, 4–5).

The ultimate question is whether or not communication technology has a worthwhile role in accelerating those information flows. However, before examining both the logic and practice of communication technology applications in agriculture, we ask a prior question: What evidence is there that investments in information produce individual or social returns greater than their cost?

There is no doubt that information flows are crucial in agricultural growth; the logic is overwhelming. But much information is passed along informally, as from parent to child or from neighbor to neighbor, or at very low marginal cost, as with the printed instructions on a fertilizer bag. In these cases and many others, individual farmers are willing to bear the cost of obtaining such information directly. They will invest time and money because the return is high. The question we must ask is more complex than whether information is of value; we must know which nonprivate investments in enhanced information flows produce a worthwhile return. In other words, when will the value of the increased output be sufficiently larger than the cost of diffusing the information so as to justify the expense? When should a government (or other institution) allocate scarce resources to organize, expand, or otherwise change currently operating information flows?

The return on information flows is best considered as we examine the specific roles for information. Information flow can be divided into three broad categories: flows to the farmer (which include education, extension, market information, and information that enables group organizing); flows to the agricultural technicians (pre- and in-service training and supervision); and flows from the field to the research and supply institutions (feedforward). We will consider the efficacy of investment in each of these areas in the following sections; however, in every case the likely return on such investments appears to be sharply conditioned by the type of agricultural resource environment in which the investment takes place.

From the time of Schultz's *Transforming Traditional Agriculture* (1964), both the theoretical and empirical literature have been largely unanimous: when a continuous stream of economically viable new technology is not available to farmers, the return on investments in information flows to farmers is small or zero. Schultz argued that traditional agriculturalists, far from being inefficient or poorly motivated (or fatalistic or noninnovative), are efficient users of available factors of production. Minimal investments in innovation reflect a low return on potential investments, not people's refusal to save. While Schultz relied on two small anthropological studies, one of an Indian village and one of a Guatemalan village, his conclusions have been supported and verified by others. As we examine evidence for returns on investment in education and information, we shall see that the availability of new technologies and the feasibility of innovations are crucial issues.

INFORMATION FLOWS TO THE FARMER

Farmer productivity, Welch (1970) argues, is substantially affected by two types of efficiency, technical efficiency and allocative efficiency, each of which may be related to flows of information. *Technical efficiency* (also called the *worker effect*) is the application of knowledge of techniques of production. The second type, *allocative efficiency*, treats the farm as a business and refers to the ability to allocate resources (for example, the ability to choose a cropping pattern, make credit arrangements, invest optimally in factors of production as crop prices change, and market the product) so as to maximize return over the long term. Nelson and Phelps (1966) add to Welch's list a third concept called *innovative effect*, which is, in some sense, a precondition to allocative efficiency. According to Chaudhri (1979), innovative effect includes the ability to decode new information, to evaluate the costs and benefits of alternative information sources, and to establish access to newly available, economically useful information.

Farmers, then, require knowledge about new inputs, new techniques of production, and how to economize in production and marketing (Wharton 1965). They also require knowledge about how to obtain these types of knowledge. What evidence is there that investment in the provision of such knowledge by institutions is worthwhile?

As Schultz and others have made clear, while a variety of ways of providing such knowledge exists, they can be divided into two broad categories: education and extension. Most careful research has focused on the impact of formal education, which, it is assumed, has its greatest impact on allocative and innovative efficiency. Less research has focused on the impact of extension, which is likely to affect the farmers' store of directly applicable knowledge and thus technical efficiency. Let us examine first the research on education and then the research on extension. There is a good deal more argument for the importance of both education and extension than there is empirical evidence.

Basic Skills Education

The theoretical literature argues that basic skills education (whether obtained in or out of school) makes six types of contributions to agricultural productivity.

First, better-educated farmers are better able to deal with, and have greater access to, external information sources. In Chaudhri's terms, they are early adopters of innovations "because their information field is superior" (1979, 3). They can get market information through correspondence or newspapers and read extension agency leaflets. Ram (quoted in Chaudhri) claims that education lowers the marginal cost of obtaining information, a point also made by Huffman (1978) and Anderson (1973). Both authors suggest that, indeed, education and extension are substitutes for one another, with Anderson arguing that educated farmers "will be able to get most of the information they need from the mass media" (p. 42). Welch (1970) showed that increased extension education reduced the productivity advantage to college education among United States farmers, a confirmation of the substitution argument.

One can also look at this enhanced information field notion from a slightly jaundiced perspective. It may be that education fosters personal relationships between farmers and similarly educated extension agents. Education may then ease access to the information giver as much as it eases access to the information.

The second value of education, in the eyes of many authors, is its positive effect on allocative ability. Schultz (1973) notes that the economic return on having a post-fourth-grade education for boys is high because of increased allocative efficiency. Education is associated with the ability to deal with the "disequilibria" endemic in operating a farm business when technology flows quickly and factor and market prices are unstable. In Wharton's language, "Mastery of the ability to think through the economic calculus is, I believe, most closely linked to the level of education" (1965, 214). Herdt (1971) agrees that education plays this role; but he suggests that only education that is directed toward developing problem-solving ability is likely to be helpful — and that, he fears, is rare in many traditional school systems.

A third value of education is its tendency to enhance farmers' "favorable attitude toward change, openness to new ideas and techniques" (Nesman et al. 1980, 45). Such innovativeness and its association with education has been the subject of literally hundreds of investigations (for summaries, see Rogers and Shoemaker 1971; Feder, Just, and Silberman 1981). It is treated with some skepticism by agricultural economists who accept Schultz's argument that profitability is a sufficient explanation for most adoption behavior, without relying on cultural variables such as innovativeness.

A fourth advantage said to accrue to better-educated farmers is the ability to perform the detailed activities associated with operating a farm business such as keeping a record of financial transactions (Chaudhri) and doing the necessary budgeting (Wharton).

Many authors have argued that a regular flow of new technology is necessary for education to affect farmer productivity, a point already made. Herdt, however, argues that the causal link runs in both directions. He suggests that a fifth consequence of increasing levels of education in a populace is that it stimulates the research institutions and extension system to provide a more rapid flow of technology. In his view, "only when an education that views technology as a means to problem-solving becomes widespread will rapidly changing technology be built into the system" (Herdt 1971, 520).

Sixth and finally, it has been argued that in a better-educated populace knowledge is more easily transmitted to all individuals in a community. This argument is made not at the individual level but at a higher level of aggregation, that of the family or the community. If the larger unit is on the average better educated, even those with less education are said to benefit because of the greater number of local channels capable of passing on new information. Nesman and colleagues report that illiterate farmers in families with a literate member are more innovative than illiterate farmers in families with no literate member.

Each of these six hypotheses details a mechanism through which education might affect agricultural productivity. Each, if confirmed, would argue for increased investment in education, including perhaps basic skills education for adults. Let us now consider the evidence. Unfortunately, there is not much helpful evidence on the mechanisms by which education affects agricultural productivity.

The best we can do is examine evidence for the overall link between education and productivity.

The empirical literature concerning the effects of education on productivity has been well summarized by Lockheed, Jamison, and Lau (1980). They present the results of thirty-one studies that estimated the economic return to four years of education (measured in various ways) on agricultural output, controlling for other variables such as land and labor input. Three generalizations may be drawn from their review:

1. On the average, there does seem to be a positive return to education: twenty-three of the thirty-one studies (75 percent) showed increased output of at least 5 percent associated with four years of education.
2. However, there is great variability in such returns, ranging from −12 percent (albeit not significantly different from zero) to more than 24 percent.
3. The variability in returns is particularly associated with the flow of technology existing in the environment of the study. Lockheed and her colleagues were able to classify twenty-three of the studies as drawing data from modernizing or nonmodernizing environments (defined by availability of certain technology). Of the sixteen studies done in modernizing environments, the mean increase in output associated with four years of education was 9 percent; for the seven data sets drawn from nonmodernizing environments the average return was about 1 percent. These results correspond closely to Schultz's predictions, summarized previously.

A great deal remains to be learned about the conditions under which education has a substantial return and about the mechanisms through which such effects occur. However, the preponderance of the evidence suggests that education can have a nontrivial impact on farmer productivity. Whether investment in education is worthwhile (from the narrow perspective of enhanced agricultural productivity) depends, of course, on the particular relation between education and output in a given environment, as well as on the local costs of education and the economic value of the increased productivity. As for adult education, it is also of some moment whether basic skills (or primary equivalent) education, which reaches out-of-school adults, has consequences similar to those of in-school education. There is no evidence on this issue; thus we can hypothesize that it is the skills and not the school-based certification that counts and that any education system that transmits such skills (whether in-school or out-of-school) will have similar consequences.

Extension
The flow of directly applicable agricultural information from central institutions to the farmer is the second type of information flow. An extension system that provides such information may enhance any of the categories of farmer efficiency previously described: technical efficiency (how and what to plant), allocative

efficiency (how to manage farm resources optimally), or innovative efficiency (how to obtain and use information). Some researchers such as Hayami and Ruttan suggest that extension activities also affect motivation to innovate as agents encourage farmers to take advantage of existing and new opportunities for improved practice.

In the economist's language, an extension system lowers the cost to the individual farmer of obtaining information, in part by shifting the cost from the individual to society, and in part through economies of scale. If the price of information is lower, more buyers will be in the market and thus more information will be diffused.

Let us turn to the evidence for returns on investment in extension. We do so, however, with great tentativeness. In our discussion of the effects of education on productivity, it was clear that context (for example, availability of technology) conditioned the effects. Also, at least one author (Herdt) argued that the type of education (rote versus problem-solving) affected the return on educational investment. If context and type are important in education, they are surely much more important in extension.

Extension, like education, may take place when there is a rapid flow of new technology and thus a great deal of information to transmit, or it may take place in an essentially static context when research institutions have produced little new technology that is adapted to local conditions. The extension system itself may be well or badly designed and operated; that is, given equal investments, two extension systems may produce very different numbers and qualities of client contact hours. Extension systems may also take on different tasks: one may provide information that enhances technical efficiency while another may enhance allocative efficiency. In Chapter 4 we shall examine current extension practice in some detail, and the great variation among systems will become evident. Thus, as we consider the evidence on the rate of return to extension investment, we do so with the knowledge that we are combining evidence from disparate systems.

There is little doubt that there is an association between contact with an extension program and innovation adoption, and an association between contact with the mass media and innovation adoption. For example, O'Sullivan (1980) found that Guatemalan farmers attended by extension agencies spent twice what nonattended farmers did on modern agricultural inputs per acre. Rogers and Shoemaker (1971) located 130 studies that showed positive associations between change-agent contact and quickness to adopt innovations and 80 studies with positive associations between mass media exposure and quickness to adopt innovations. But these associational data tell us little. We need to know (1) that such associations reflect a causal process; (2) that access to information and not some other aspect of extension contact, such as access to credit, made the difference; and (3) that the effects on rate of adoption translate into effects on productivity such that the rates of return to extension expenditures are worthwhile. Locating studies that satisfy these conditions has proved to be difficult.

Evidence about the effects of extension comes from three sources: (1) studies of the association between individual farmer contact with extension services or media believed to carry extension messages and innovations adopted (or productivity); (2) studies of aggregate associations between investment in extension and agricultural production, with either nations or districts within nations serving as analysis units; and (3) studies of the effects of particular extension programs, which are almost always comparative studies of numbers of recommended innovations adopted among those exposed and those not (or not yet) exposed to the extension program.

Studies of Individuals. There is ample evidence that extension agent contact and media exposure are associated with improved farming practices and outcomes in at least some circumstances. Nonetheless, little of that data justifies investment in extension in order to improve information flows to the farmer. The data provide no useful evidence for or against such investment. We review it briefly here and then explain our reluctance to rely on such data.

We have cited evidence that change-agent contact and media exposure are associated with adoption of innovations. In many but not all cases, those associations hold up even when other variables, such as socioeconomic status or land size, which might suggest that causal inference from such associations is spurious, are controlled (Roy et al. 1969; O'Sullivan 1980). Beyond that, when adoption of innovations is replaced by farm productivity as the criterion variable, in most cases extension contact is still positively associated with output. In fifteen of the seventeen studies reviewed by Orivel (1981) and Lockheed and associates (1980), the extension/output relation is positive, and in seven of those studies that relationship is significantly different from zero. Thus extension contact seems not only to predict adoption of innovations, but also with some frequency, improvements in productivity. Yet, when viewed as evidence justifying investment in extension systems to enhance information flows to the farmer, this data is fundamentally flawed.

First, these studies do not, as a group, make it clear what aspect of extension affects innovativeness or productivity. As we have noted, most measures of extension worker contact are not merely measures of information flow, the concept of interest to us, but are also measures of, among other things, access to credit and to sources of agricultural inputs. We cannot make inferences about information effects of extension worker contact unless we can control for the effects of these other roles. This has not been done in most of these studies.

There is a similar problem in the studies of mass media effects on agricultural outcomes. Some agricultural communication projects make specific use of media; we examine evidence derived from those projects in the section below on project-based evidence. Most studies, however, merely show an association between general media exposure (most often radio listening) and adoption of innovation. Even if such associations are nonspurious (see Contreras 1980), defining what aspect of the media exposure had such effects is problematic. Agricultural programming (including didactic programs, but also weather forecasts and market price lists) makes up only a small part of what is available. At least some theories of media effect suggest alternative paths through which media exposure might encourage improved agricultural practice (see Inkeles and Smith 1974; or Rogers and Svenning 1969; both argue that the mass media are a school for modern values). Thus even unambiguous evidence that media use affects agricultural productivity would not directly justify increases in agricultural programming on radio. We would need to isolate agricultural programming effects from general effects, just as we need to isolate extension-agent information effects from the effects of extension-agent credit access.

A second problem relates only to those studies that depend on adoption of innovations as their criterion variable. Some innovations recommended by extension agents enhance productivity only in minor ways or require complementary practice changes to have nontrivial effects. For example, O'Sullivan found that adoption of some innovations (maintaining a compost pile, spacing of seeds, and other practice changes that entailed minimal cash commitments on the part of the farmer) had little direct effect on productivity, while others (fertilizer use, insecticide use, and other practices that required cash) had relatively large effects. Yet in a typical study of the effects of extension on innovation, a summary index of innovations adopted is the criterion variable; and it is quite possible that the association between extension contact and adoption speaks to change in practices that do not affect productivity.

The third major issue is the lack of data about worthwhile rates of return to extension. Let us assume that in at least some circumstances, the diffusion of extension-based information has a real effect on adoption of innovation and on productivity. Clearly, that is not enough to know. If $100 had to be spent on extension for each $10 increase in productivity, the expense would scarcely be justified. Such investments are justified only when the productive value of the outcome achieved through extension inputs implies a rate of return comparable to that achieved through alternative investment opportunities.

In fact, when we look at the data from these individual-level studies, we see that a rate of return has been calculated only rarely. And in six of the seven cases where it has been (based on data provided in Lockheed et al. 1980), the confidence band around the benefit-cost ratios includes a possible benefit-cost ratio of less than one, suggesting that we cannot reject the hypothesis that costs may be larger than benefits.

So far we have raised issues that cast doubt on the quality of the evidence for positive effects of extension. If observed associations may overestimate the effects of extension, they may also systematically underestimate them. Two flaws in typical extension studies may produce such a downward bias. First, typically, individual exposure to extension-generated information is estimated by reported contacts with extension agents. Yet that measurement strategy contradicts one of the basic underpinnings of developing country extension (albeit one frequently challenged): that the effects of extension-agent contact diffuse from the contacted farmer to other farmers in the social network. Those farmers reached by the so-called two-step flow would not report extension-agent contact, yet they might have been affected by that contact. The result would be an attenuation of the relation between extension-agent contact and productivity, and thus an underestimate of extension's consequences. (Only in Jamison and Lau's Thai study [cited in Lockheed et al.] is this problem resolved. It contrasts farmers living in villages with and without extension services available, rather than farmers within a given village with and without extension contact.)

In a related discussion, Huffman (1978) notes that private diffusion expenditures (those paid by individuals or commercial entities) may not be incorporated in studies that focus on contact with government-paid extension agents. However, such privately financed extension contact may also affect productivity. Depending on the association of private expenditure with public expenditure, the estimates of public expenditure effects may be biased upward or downward. If the same farmers tend to have contact with both private and public extension services, then the estimates of rates of return attributed to public extension alone are too high. If, in contrast, better-off farmers ignore the public system for a private one and, therefore, appear as individuals with little extension contact but good productivity in a study of the public system, such a study is likely to underestimate the return to public extension.

The second issue whose consequences are likely to lead to a false inference of no effect concerns the time distribution of effects. Most sets of data associate current contact with extension agents with current productivity. Yet the association introduces two misleading factors into the calculation of extension consequences. It is not necessarily true that current contact correlates perfectly with previous contact. It is possible that, averaged over a number of years, estimates of individual contact with extension agents would be different from the data gathered on a single year's contacts. If the typical pattern is followed, there would be a tendency for those described as lower or higher than the average on the basis of a single year's data to appear closer to the average if multiple-year data are averaged. This phenomenon would result in observed associations based on single-year data underestimating associations based on multiyear estimates of contact.

A second time-related subissue applies specifically to those studies that estimate a rate of return. It is our assumption that the effects of extension contacts, even on the individual farmer who is contacted, are not all produced in the year of the contacts. For example, diffusion theory (Rogers 1983) suggests that farmers may try out a new seed variety on a small part of their land one year and adopt it for all their acreage the following year if its yield meets expectations. The extension contacts are likely to take place the first year, but the increase in productivity will appear the following year. A study that looks only at current contacts and productivity, and assumes no time lag in effects, will underestimate the actual association. Amortization of current extension expenditures over the entire period of their effects (future as well as present) and cumulation of the (appropriately discounted) value of the future effects are likely to improve benefit-cost ratios. (Huffman suggests that the biases lent by such time effects are small, since they are likely to be counterbalanced by the failure to include previous years' costs of extension in accounting for current effects.)

An additional underestimation of effects is likely to result from the use of a single equation to capture all of the consequences of extension. Huffman suggests that coefficients based on equations that include both input factors and extension as simultaneous predictors of productivity ignore the indirect effects of extension on productivity through its effects on input factors. If extension effects on productivity are actually the result of extension effects leading farmers to increased expenditure on seed or fertilizer, those effects are likely to be lost.

To summarize, a useful study of the effects of extension on productivity should (1) introduce controls for third variables that might explain the bivariate association between contact and productivity, (2) allow estimation of a rate of return to extension outlays (or at least allow the estimation of productivity gains that can be compared with separately estimated extension costs across different environments), (3) take into account the probability that extension effects extend beyond the contacted farmer, and (4) respect the effects of time lags of extension consequences. None of the studies we have located satisfies these conditions.

Aggregate Studies. A second small group of studies makes use of data about extension investments aggregated by country, or region within country, and associates those data with similarly aggregated estimates of agricultural product. They are then able to make estimates of rates of return to extension expenditures, controlling for other sources of agricultural productivity. A half-dozen studies done in the United States led Huffman to conclude that "the returns to extension, at least in the United States, are modest or better" (1978, 969). We found only one study, Evenson and Jha (1973), that used cross-regional aggregate data to estimate the rate of return to extension investment in a developing country. They estimated a productivity function for fifteen Indian states over three time periods. They measured the maturity of a state's extension system, the expenditure on agricultural research within that state and other states with similar climates, agricultural output, and other variables. Overall, they found the return on research investment to be very high, the direct effects of extension investment minimal, and the interaction of extension and research investment to be positive. These findings translate into a moderate rate of return to extension but only if a state invests in research also.

While this study is of substantial interest, it suffers inevitably from some of the same flaws that affected the individual studies previously described. The most important of these is its failure to differentiate the information diffusion functions of extension from other functions — particularly that of serving as a conduit for inputs (such as seeds and fertilizer) and credit.

Studies of Particular Projects. Almost all of the previous studies examined effects of normal, ongoing extension activities. A final group of studies comes from the evaluation of projects designed to explore new extension (or agricultural development) approaches. We consider these in detail in subsequent sections.

By and large, such evaluations do not show consistent evidence of increased productivity or reasonable rates of return, almost always because no attempt was made to estimate such statistics. When strong evidence of improvement is presented, it is impossible to separate the effects of extension, per se, from the effects of the complementary institutional changes (credit availability, new seeds, enhanced marketing possibilities) that accompany improvements in extension in apparently successful projects.

FACTOR AND MARKET PRICE INFORMATION

Education and extension are said to provide the farmer with the capacity to manage a farm optimally — both in the sense of maximizing productivity and in the sense of being responsive to changing factor prices and market prices for crops. The latter depends in turn on farmers having information about factor costs and, if they are commercial farmers, market prices. The flow of factor and market price information to the farmer is the third of those flows of information that a public agency might consider enhancing. Our question is, Would it pay off to invest in such things as radio reports of prices that improve the recency and amount of information farmers now have?

Most of this section concentrates on exploring the conceptual issues surrounding this question; applicable evidence is hard to find. The first question we must ask is whether or not existing information systems leave farmers substantially ignorant of factor and market prices. There are, after all, many informal systems for the diffusion of such information, and farmers certainly make use of them. Is the gap very large between what farmers estimate those prices to be and what they actually are? A very large gap in this case would imply that if farmers knew the true prices, they would reap an economic advantage by allocating their farm resources differently.

Next, if one assumes that such large inaccuracies in price information exist, would improved access to information make a difference in the farmers' behavior? While this query may seem to question the assumption of the farmers' economic rationality so strongly endorsed earlier, it need not. Some common circumstances among LDC farmers make economically rational behavior infeasible. Let us use the example of the farmers who market crops through middlemen. It is sometimes claimed that farmers sell at lower prices than the market would permit, in part because they are not aware of what actual market prices are. For the sake of the example, one can assume (although empirical evidence is lacking and would be required) that farmers in this circumstance inaccurately perceive market prices; they do not know what proportion of the eventual sales price they actually receive. Next, assume that a daily market price radio broadcast achieved perfect price knowledge for farmers. Is it the case that the farmers' share of market value will increase? Not necessarily. Farmers may be locked into a sales arrangement (perhaps negotiated in return for credit to buy inputs) that requires sales at fixed, nonmarket prices. Similarly, the risks and costs (in time or money) of alternative sales arrangements may absorb no less of the farmers' profits than do the middlemen.

Better knowledge of factor prices also may not translate to higher farm profits if farmers lack the flexibility to respond. For example, soy beans may produce a greater return in a given year than corn, and farmers responding to prices ought to plant accordingly; but if the farmers do not know how to plant soy, or if credit is unavailable at short notice, they will pass up the opportunity. Their environment (and one need not refer to psychological or cultural inflexibility) does not permit responsiveness to rapidly changing price signals. It may be that the speed at which their natural diffusion networks provide market and factor price information corresponds to the farmer's degree of flexibility in adapting farming decisions. They find out what they need to know, and what they do not know they probably would not have used anyway.

We then have three alternative formulations: farmers have an accurate knowledge of factor and market prices; farmers lack such knowledge but could not use it if they had it; and farmers lack such knowledge and would improve their profits if they had it. Only the third suggests that investment in enhanced price information systems would be productive — and then only if the benefits were greater than the cost. What does the evidence indicate? Which of the three circumstances describes best the circumstances of LDC farmers? Or more realistically, How many farmers (and what types of farmers) fall into each category?

To answer these questions, we have two somewhat indirect types of evidence. First, despite some controversy, there is "ample evidence. . .that subsistence farmers adjust their production in response to price changes" (Toquero et al. 1975, 705; Behrman 1967; Krishna 1967). In Behrman's estimation, those responses are "of the same order of magnitude as those which have been reported for higher income customers" (p. 47). This is evidence that at least some of the variation in market price is returned to the farmer — otherwise no responsiveness could be expected. However, this clearly does not guarantee that farmers capture their full fair share — if that is defined as the market price less the actual value of marketing services. It could be that as prices increase, the middleman takes a larger absolute amount of the price per unit, even though the actual marketing cost per unit remains unchanged.

Hayami and Ruttan (1971) argue that the strongest test of the hypothesis that farmers are underpaid comes from a comparison of farm and market prices over time or across regions for a given crop. If the middlemen are in fact taking a share that reflects their actual marketing costs and those marketing costs do not change with the price of the crop, then the relationship between farm prices and market prices should be linear. If, in contrast, marketers increase their charges as market prices go up (although their costs remain constant), then the association between farm price and market price should be nonlinear.

According to Hayami and Ruttan, four studies (Ruttan 1969, in the Philippines; Allen 1959, in East Pakistan; Behrman 1968, in Thailand; and Lele 1967, in India) have taken this approach and found essentially a linear relation between farm and market prices. That data is "inconsistent with the hypothsis that middlemen profit by widening the margin between farmers and consumers during periods when retail prices are relatively high" (Hayami and Ruttan 1971, 266).

McDowell (n.d.), however, has reassessed these results and is skeptical about their definitiveness. He notes that these studies, in some cases, examine not farm-to-market prices but primary market to terminal market prices. He claims that, in fact, there is often substantial deviation from linearity representing possible middleman profiteering, but which is ignored in the Hayami and Ruttan synthesis.

Even Hayami and Ruttan admit that the commodity markets studied were characterized by rather slow growth in production and demand. In situations of rapid change, expectations of a linear relation might be unreasonable, either because the information system failed to communicate price signals between consumers and producers, or because the marketing systems were not able to expand rapidly enough to maintain perfect competition among marketers — so that the price of marketing services increased.

Hayami and Ruttan's analyses suggest that many LDC farmers fit the first of the three formulations — they have a reasonable knowledge of factor and market prices (although the reported data deal only with market prices). McDowell is less convinced and suggests that the available evidence is inconsistent and often indirect. In his view, the potential for market and factor information cannot be ruled out. Given either view, investments in enhanced information systems must await the location of situations where farmers are in fact ill-informed and, because of that poor information, are unable to reap the full benefit of their farm resources.

INFORMATION FLOWS TO DEVELOP
FARMER ORGANIZATION

In the view of some, the development of farmer organizations is essential to agricultural development. Esman (1974) articulates the logic of this argument most clearly. Given the shortage of extension agents, the mass of individual farmers cannot now, and will not in the future, be reached directly. In contrast, farmers' organizations can serve as points of diffusion, muliplying the effects of agents. In addition, if innovations are adopted by groups rather than by individuals, the sense of uncertainty and risk is likely to be reduced. However, the functions of organization are broader in Esman's view. Local adaptation of agricultural advice is essential; yet individual farmers are not effective in articulating specific local needs. That feedback process, through which local needs guide the activities undertaken by agricultural institutions, is enhanced potentially by the existence of farmers' organizations, which as "collectivities. . . can articulate needs which the individual small farmer cannot" (p. 74).

Farmers' organizations, according to Esman, can also contribute to integrating the activities of credit, extension, and irrigation agencies so as to reduce the "multiple and even conflicting advice" that an individual farmer may face (1974, 74). Finally, as an organized political force, farmers may more successfully compete for scarce resources. For the moment we are not concerned as to whether (or under what circumstances) Esman's hypothesis about the effects of organizing is correct. The issue is whether externally generated information flows are likely to help local organizations develop.

No doubt there is a paradox in the formulation of that question and its linking of external actions and local group development. After all, the value of local groups is their ability to articulate and fight for local needs independently of outside control. Nonetheless, despite the legitimate demand for local participation and for respect of local needs, most who endorse local organization see a central role for outsiders in stimulating the development of such organizations.

The criteria for judging the efficacy of externally generated information in stimulating local organizations are more elusive than for other types of information. No longer are enhanced productivity or increased agricultural income available as immediately expected outcomes. We must look for evidence of effective organization — organization that lasts for more than a brief time, that undertakes specific development activity, that draws upon and articulates local interests, and that is able to engage competing interests in the struggle for scarce resources. The extent to which an organization represents the range of interest in its area rather than the interests of but one local stratum, perhaps at the cost of others, is also a criterion for evaluation. Ideally, local organizations become substantially independent of (although perhaps allied with) the external organizations that provided their original impetus.

In subsequent sections, we shall describe a number of projects, using communication technology or not, that have attempted to create local organizations, generally as part of a program with specific agricultural development objectives. It is, however, beyond the scope of this presentation to attempt a systematic evaluation of efforts to generate local organizations.

INFORMATION FLOWS TO AGRICULTURAL TECHNICIANS

The evidence for the efficacy of extension activities is not clear-cut. In this section, however, we shall assume that extension is sometimes worthwhile, and that active agents in the field are the most likely channels for such extension activity. In that case, information that flows to the extension agent may be of no less importance than information that flows from the agent to the farmer. That information can be of many types.

There is information about new seeds or fertilizers and about new techniques of farming. In our earlier discussion, we pointed to the consensus among many scholars that extension is of value only if there is a constant flow of new technology to be adopted. If there is such a flow, it is clear that extension agents need constant in-service training in order to be able to offer up-to-date advice. In situations where a variety of crops are being sown, and the expertise of local agents is limited, information from subject-matter specialists may be particularly important.

Other information flows provide supervision and psychological support for extension agents. Direct and continuous contact between supervisors and agents, according to Mosher (1978) and Benor and Harrison (1977), supports and monitors agents as they carry out expected work activities on the appropriate schedule. It enables organization of in-service training activities and permits changes in the schedule of activities if required (for example, the urgent diffusion of techniques to fight an unexpected plant disease). At the same time, the maintenance of an information flow between a field agent and a central office may serve the psychological needs of the agent. The agent, often from another area and certainly trained in the city, may feel isolated. The constant flow of information may reduce this sense of isolation. One might expect better day-to-day motivation and lower turnover among agents if this hypothesis is correct.

We have not found studies that evaluate the outcome of such information flows (that is, pre-service and in-service training and support) in isolation from the rest of an extension system. The logic for some form of information support to agents is quite strong; nonetheless, we would wish to know the value of particular levels and methods of such support (it can vary from a very low-cost system of twice-yearly supervisory visits to a costly system of biweekly training seminars and daily two-way radio communication).

INFORMATION FLOWS FROM FARMERS

The argument for enhanced flows of information to farmers depends on the assumption that normal communication systems will be insufficient to diffuse information about economically useful technology. Many authors are skeptical about this assumption; they argue that farmers are indeed responsive to economic signals and will obtain information that they can use. However, while farmers may be sensitive to the signals from the agricultural institutions with which they deal, there is substantial doubt as to whether the opposite is true. A constant flow of new technology well adapted to a microgeographical region is said to be a necessary stimulus to productivity growth. However, the proper development and adaptation of technology may require an information flow from farmer to research institution that is not often realized.

Mosher, Hayami, and Ruttan, and Axinn and Thorat, among many others, argue that effective links among the components of the agricultural system (production, supply, marketing, extension) are crucial to efficient operation. In

Axinn and Thorat's language, "the crucial input that converts the farmer from peasant to scientific business manager, that converts the nation from food deficit to food exporter...is the integration of research and education with...supply, with production, and with marketing" (1972, 6). Such integration requires both effective communication and receptiveness to the message received.

McDermott argues that one of the most important activities of the United States extension system was "maintaining relevance in the research and teaching functions of the agricultural colleges" (1971, 153). The county agents in the field, by constantly "feeding forward" the needs of the farmers, provide guidance to the research institutions. However, in much of the developing world, extension agents reach only a small proportion of the farmers; and the farmers they do reach are generally advantaged with greater resources and with a commercial orientation (Roling et al. 1976; O'Sullivan 1980). The agents will not be able to transmit the requirements of subsistence farmers if they are not in regular contact with them. Because the agents themselves may also be administratively isolated from research institutions, no channel of communication may be available. This is particularly likely if research activities are substantially centralized. Thus, despite widespread agreement that a link between farmer and research institution is essential, there may not be such a link.

Even if there is such a link, it may be that research institutions do not respond to the relayed demands. In the view of many authors, individual farmers are entrepreneurs who maximize profits and who are thus likely to respond to price signals. Research institutions, in contrast, are most often public institutions with limited resources to allocate and many demands on their capacity. Hayami and Ruttan argue that efficient information links should assure "that demand and supply of products and factors produce price signals that will efficiently guide research and the process of innovation down an appropriate local path." But, as Schuh and Tollini state, "there are little by way of market signals to allocate research resources" (1979, 2).

Hayami and Ruttan admit that, in the case of public research institutions, they assume that public benefits will motivate an institution. Critics like Ashby and her colleagues (1978) take a somewhat skeptical view of this assumption. They argue that farmers with larger holdings are actively opposed to improvements among subsistence farmers and are likely to oppose successfully research directed toward their needs. Given the apparent high rates of return to research (Boyce and Evenson 1975; Orivel 1981), there has clearly been a history of underinvestment in research. Such underinvestment is consistent with the view of Ashby and her colleagues.

Even without adopting a rich-farmer versus poor-farmer conflict perspective, one can see other motivations, besides that of maximum public benefit, playing some role in guiding research institutions. For example, scholarly prestige, often the coin most sought by researchers, may be tied to research publishable in international circles as opposed to research that produces the largest income streams locally. Also, given that public benefit is in fact difficult to estimate (Schuh and Tollini 1979), even if researchers were interested in maximizing such outcomes, it would be difficult to know how to assign resources.

As we consider whether or not investment in information flows from the farmer to the agricultural institutions is likely to improve efficiency and equity in the agricultural sector, we must bring these alternative perspectives to bear. Is it true that research and other institutions are insufficiently responsive to farmers' needs? If so, what are useful ways of enhancing farmer influence on the institutions that serve them? Are the obstacles essentially technical failures in communication? In this case, a strategy for gathering information more efficiently (perhaps through sampling farmers of different strata) is required. Or are the problems political? In this case, efficient transmission of farmers' requirements must be supplemented by effective aggregation of political interests so as to influence the allocation of resources. Evidence on whether or not formal programs designed to enhance feedforward affect the activities of research institutions to the benefit of farmers has not been found. As with efforts to improve technical support and training, the few examples of such projects have been directed toward other activities and purposes also. They will be discussed in a subsequent chapter.

We have described six types of information flows — each a candidate to be enhanced by investment: basic skills education, extension, market information, organizing information, technical support training, and feedforward. Although, for at least several of these, there has been a long history of investment, the efficiency of such investment is open to question. This partly reflects negative evidence or evidence of uncertain relevance; but it mostly reflects a lack of evidence altogether. Relying on what we have seen thus far, we can conclude:

1. that education has some positive consequences when new technology is available;
2. that the rate of return to extension is sometimes positive but cannot be confidently assigned to the information-diffusion function rather than other functions of extension;
3. that there is unclear evidence as to whether farmers are currently ignorant of factor or market prices when it would be to their advantage to be knowledgeable; and
4. that we have little evidence, beyond the appeal of the arguments themselves, of the value of investment in information for group organization, for field agent support, or for influencing research institutions.

We cannot, then, speak very confidently based on the data reviewed thus far. The evidence drawn from research not closely tied to specific programs cannot give us definitive answers about the value of investments in information. In the next chapters, while still seeking evidence about the value of information, we turn to evidence from specific projects. That evidence will help us to understand how projects designed to affect one or more of these information flows operate and, in some cases, give us some evidence about outcomes. However, we will find ourselves less able to make general statements about the utility of investments in information than we would have been had the more general data presented in this section borne fruit.

Chapter Four

Information Programs without Communication Technology

In this chapter, we shall review agricultural information approaches that do not depend heavily on communication technology. Our review is not comprehensive; a number of sources provide detailed reviews (Coombs and Ahmed 1974; Morss et al. 1976; Rice 1974; ECA-FAO 1971). Instead, we classify and illustrate the types of programs that have been undertaken and draw from them a list of crucial problems that information programs must solve if they are to be successful. We use that material as background to the subsequent and more detailed exploration of communication technology programs and their potential role for resolving the crucial problems.

Two points about the organization of this chapter will become apparent. We have ignored projects that provide basic skills education to farmers unless they are part of a broader agricultural project. Secondly, we do not organize the section by types of information flows addressed. In almost every case, the projects considered are engaged primarily in extension activities, and any other functions they serve are integrated into the central extension activity. A division by information function, with individual projects described under more than one heading, would have ignored the systematic nature of these programs.

Each project is discussed in terms of degree of success or failure, obstacles to success, and factors that appear to reduce the possibility of failure. Yet there is no strong evidence that any form of extension activity (or, for that matter, any investment in information flows except for basic education) is cost beneficial. It might seem then to be specious to talk about the relative utility of alternative approaches to enhancing information flows when little evidence exists that enhanced information flows help in any formulation. It is done (albeit with some trepidation) for two reasons. First, the evidence does not, in most cases, deny the effectiveness of extension investments; rather it is inadequate to resolve the issue. Failure to find evidence of success may reflect the failure of extension as a concept, the failure of the extension strategy studied, the failure of the strategy in the particular agricultural context (for example, the extent to which new technology is available), the failure to realize the strategy adequately, or the failure to gather appropriate evidence for valid judgments to be made. In general, the evidence we have does not allow us to distinguish among these explanations.

Second, we think it justified to discuss alternative strategies of enhanced information flow because almost everyone who writes about the subject says it is useful. Even the harshest critics of traditional extension activities (Schultz, Rice, and Coombs and Ahmed) unequivocally state that farmer information programs are worthwhile under the right circumstances: generally if they take place when there is a good deal of new technology being generated, and if they are integrated with other elements of what Mosher (1969) calls a "Progressive Rural Structure." Almost all governments and most international aid agencies support information activities either in isolation or in association with integrated agricultural programs (Boyce and Evenson 1975). Farmers need to know, and most writers and field workers believe, that deliberate efforts to accelerate the diffusion process (even if market incentives are both a necessary condition and crucial impetus for that diffusion) are justified. Quantitative evidence on the subject is to be preferred, but until it is available one can only accept the field's assumption: agricultural information programs would be valuable if they could be done right. Just what doing them right means, and the difficulties of realizing such an ideal model, will become clear as we discuss what has been done in the past.

Coombs and Ahmed describe three approaches to agricultural information: conventional extension, self-help community development, and integrated agricultural development. With some strain these categories match the types of information programs described in other sources also (cf. ECA-FAO 1971; Rice 1974). We describe each of those and then look separately at a fourth type of program, the Training and Visit System, sponsored by the World Bank.

CONVENTIONAL EXTENSION

Much of the literature describing LDC activities in extension dates from the mid-1970s. If what is written there still holds, conventional extension is virtually universal and is sometimes complemented by the other strategies described below. Rice (1974) describes Latin American extension services as almost always the product of United States technical assistance of the 1950s and early 1960s. Elsewhere, if not the result of direct intervention, "in most cases [extension programs] have been inspired by the extension program of the United States" (Mosher 1976, 133). However, neither intervention nor inspiration has produced close imitations of the United States model. Rice describes the typical Latin American system as follows:

> In general what one finds in these countries is an entity called the *división de extensión agrícola* within the directorate of agriculture, one of the major units of the ministry of agriculture and livestock. The *división* has a director and a deputy, and, if it is in a large country, several area supervisors of agencies. There is also a national supervisor for home economics, another for rural youth programs, and another for information and visual aids. There will be a small unit of subject matter specialists at

headquarters, a unit that often numbers no more than four or five, including an agronomist, a livestock specialist, a tropical fruit man, etc.

In the field one finds a number of *agencias*, probably one for each province or whatever the third largest geographic administrative unit is called (similar to counties in the U.S.). The agency is run by an agent and a male secretary. There is usually an assistant agent who handles club work. In about half the agencies one finds a home economist. The agency staff shares a common jeep, which is five years old and past retirement age. The agent and his staff have some pamphlets to give away, but they have little or no fertilizer, seed or credit to offer the farmer. The agent, the assistant agent and the home economist are in the field about seventy percent of the time, often in the same village (they have to travel together) but rarely working with the same family unit. They have little contact with other agricultural professionals resident in the same town, for example the credit agents and fertilizer salesmen, and they stay away from the local research station, if there is one, unless that is where the ministry keeps the gasoline it supplies for all ministry vehicles.

A large part of the time spent in the office is devoted to reports, of which there are many, covering different aspects of the schedule. There are weekly and monthly status reports, and annual summaries of them showing where the staff has been and what they have been doing. There are monthly, quarterly and annual plans. There are vehicle use forms, expenditure forms, etc. The secretary types them up and sends them to the supervisor (1974, 90–91).

Coombs and Ahmed's description of the Kenyan and Nigerian services and the ECA-FAO's description of other East African programs are essentially consistent with Rice's description of Latin American services.

The extension agent's role in that description was that of diffuser of available information. It was assumed that there was extant valuable technology, and the main task was to educate farmers in its application. As Coombs and Ahmed point out, "few extensionists any longer hold strictly to this view" (1974, 24); but "in practice both the extension and training approaches seem to operate on the assumption [that] useful knowledge flows mainly in one direction: from outside specialists to the rural clienteles" (p.25). While often a two-way flow of information is assumed to exist between the agents and farmers and the research agencies, the strong bureaucratic isolation of the two services and the lack of any formal mechanism for feedforward means that it rarely occurs.

Educational methods utilized by agents vary, of course, but the essential elements appear and reappear in almost every descriptive report and in guides to extension (Mosher 1978; Fisher et al. 1968; Maunder 1972). They include individual approaches (farm visits or office contacts), group methods (result and method demonstrations, group meetings, tours, and farmer's field days), and mass media (visual aids, pamphlets, posters, radio). In addition, and in particular for African extension services, the agent's direct work is supplemented by local training centers. A Kenyan farmer training center typically gives one-week courses "tending to concentrate on single aspects of cash crop production or animal husbandry" (Coombs and Ahmed 1974, 37).

Conventional extension, while it remains the most commonly implemented farmer information strategy, is almost universally criticized by outside reviewers (Coombs and Ahmed 1974; Morss et al. 1976; ECA-FAO 1971; Rice 1974; Axinn and Thorat 1972). We shall review some themes of those critiques, organizing them by issue, into four categories: reach, appropriate recommendations, training, and long-term efficacy. Each of these, first analyzed as a typical problem of conventional extension, provides a springboard for the examination of alternative approaches to farmer information which may be seen as attempts to resolve one or more of these problems.

Audience Reach

It is difficult to define an ideal extension-agent-to-farming-household ratio. While the FAO chose 500 farm families per agent "as a minimum standard," other authorities have made other choices (Rice 1974, 121). The USAID Nigeria Saturation project (Nelson and Kazungu 1973) sought one worker per 1,800 farmers. Mosher argued that if "all of the diffusion of improved practices depended on extension workers, a ratio of about 400 farmers to one extension worker would be the effective limit" (1969, 121). However, in his recommendation for an ideal "Progressive Rural Structure," he chose 1,200 farmers to one worker, assuming that farmer-to-farmer diffusion would be important. By 1970 the Unites States maintained a ratio of 500 farmers per agricultural extension agent, an improvement from a ratio of 1,500 farms per agent thirty years before (Rogers, Eveland, and Bean 1976, 166). Even the 500-to-1 figure, we shall see, may not represent effective saturation. Obviously, the ideal farmer-to-agent ratio can be specified only in terms of the local context: what extent of contact is required to have any impact, the nature of the changes that are to be recommended, how geographically separated farmers are, the efficacy of farmer-to-farmer diffusion networks, and other factors.

What is actually realized, with regard to farmer-to-agent ratios, is extraordinarily variable. The ECA-FAO report, using 1968 data, reported between 200 and 400 farm families per agent in Kenya, Zambia, and the Malagasy Republic, but 14,000 families per agent in Somalia, and 27,000 per agent in Ethiopia. South Korea, as reported in Coombs and Ahmed, had about 425 farm families per extension worker in 1971, a number maintained through 1974 (Boyce and Evenson 1975), while India's 56,000 village-level workers (1965 data from Boyce and Evenson) were each assigned more than 1,000 families spread over ten villages (Coombs and Ahmed 1974). The Latin American data is in less accessible form; but by combining estimates from Rice, Boyce and Evenson, and the World Bank and assuming that there is one farm household for every ten rural persons, we can make some estimates. As of 1970, ratios varied from perhaps 600 families per agent in Brazil and 1,100 families per agent in Costa Rica to 3,700 families per agent in Bolivia.

While families per agent is the best measure of reach, it is inadequate. It does not reflect the distribution of agents to the farming population. O'Sullivan,

Roling, and others have documented the tendency for agents to help better-off farmers, leaving subsistence farmers on their own. Also, countries may concentrate available resources in particular regions (as India did with its Intensive Agricultural District Program), or they may concentrate on particular (often export) crops (as Colombia does for its coffee industry) (Rice 1974, 368).

Also, knowing how many agents there are indicates nothing about the quality of the work they do or how much of their time is spent on agriculture (or particularly on farmer information tasks). In the United States, virtually every agent holds a bachelor's degree in agronomy. In contrast, in South Korea's Office of Rural Development, which Coombs and Ahmed point to as a sophisticated version of conventional extension, only 10 percent of the agents have college training. In Senegal, the only requirement for service as an extension agent is "some formal education." Rice suggests that university-trained extensionists are also rare in most of Latin America. We do not want to argue that a college agronomy degree is a necessary or a sufficient condition for quality extension service. However, it is an indication of the level of substantive sophistication the workers are likely to bring to the field, and thus an indicator of their ability to work autonomously.

In many countries, extension agents, along with primary school teachers, may be the only government representatives who penetrate deeply into rural areas. The temptation is great to add many other functions to their farmer education responsibilities. Some do other work in the agricultural sector: regulatory functions, which are particularly common in Africa (ECA-FAO); seed, credit, and fertilizer distribution; organization and supervision of 4-H clubs; and agricultural censuses. In some places, extension workers fill many roles and functions and are responsible for all community development work. In India's Community Development Program, which sponsored village-level workers throughout the country, agricultural extension made up only 40 percent of the activity of those workers. The ratio of 1,000 families per worker cited previously is therefore misleading and should have been 1,000 families per 0.4 workers, or 2,500 families per worker.

Whether the ratio be 500 or 1,500 or 5,000 to one worker, the number of farmers actually reached individually is going to be far less. Fisher and his colleagues offer a telling calculation in their manual *Agricultural Extension Training* (1968). Working in Kenya, they found that agents could make individual farm visits at the rate of two per day. Assuming 300 work days per year, a maximum of 600 visits could be realized. Again assuming each farmer concerned must be seen at least once a month, the maximum number of farmers to be seen by a single agent is about 50. If an agent visited each home every two months, a total of 100 farms might be covered. These numbers are consistent with descriptions of individual agent activity in Latin America found by Rice (1974, 340).

Obviously, extension agents must assume a very large multiplier effect, with many unreached farmers imitating farmers actually helped by agents; or agents must use methods that enable them to reach many more farmers simultaneously.

It is no surprise that Morss and his colleagues conclude, "[T]here will never be sufficient numbers of highly trained agronomists and agriculture extensionists to allow the kind of frequency of supervision necessary for complex agricultural change" (1976, 2:131). If they are right, it will not be because governments have been unwilling to increase their extension expenditures. Conventional extension systems are expensive. Perraton and colleagues (1983) estimate the costs in Malawi to be $21 per farmer contact, for a conventional extension system that reaches 10 percent of the farm population.

From 1959 to 1974, there was a two- to threefold increase among the poorest countries in the proportion of the value of their agricultural product devoted to extension. Table 4.1 displays not only the extraordinary relative increases of the poorest countries but also indicates that the poor countries are spending relatively more than wealthier countries for their extension activities. For example, those countries whose per capita income was less than $150 spent nearly 2 percent of the value of their agricultural product on extension, while wealthier nations (per capita income greater than $1,750) spent only 0.6 percent. In contrast to extension advocates like Benor and Harrison (1977), who argue that the returns on sharply expanded extension services easily justify the investment, Boyce and Evenson (1975) note that poor countries, relative to wealthy countries, are already underinvesting in research compared to extension, and returns could be higher if they shifted toward research. Since there is inadequate data on the returns on each type of investment, the issue can only be opened here. However, given the already high levels of investment in extension among poor countries, it is difficult to imagine sharp increases in extension unless the service is directly financed through a share of the increased income it produces.

Appropriate Recommendations

Conventional extension held a central assumption: that the major obstacle to improvement in farmer productivity was farmer knowledge and attitude. If only the information were diffused and known technology adopted, all would be well. Few would argue such a proposition now. In Mosher's words, extension systems in the United States (which were the model for many developing countries) took

TABLE 4.1. Extension and Research Expenditures as a Percent of the Value of Agricultural Product by Per-capita Income Group

Income Group	Research Expenditure				Extension Expenditure			
	1959	*1965*	*1971*	*1974*	*1959*	*1965*	*1971*	*1974*
I More than $1,750	.79	1.09	1.44	1.48	.45	.52	.61	.60
II $1,001–$1,750	.80	1.38	1.76	1.83	.17	.22	.33	.31
III $401–$1,001	.45	.67	.86	.92	.26	.40	.46	.40
IV $150–$400	.33	.53	.71	.84	.67	.99	1.44	1.59
V Less than $150	.29	.64	.86	.88	.57	1.04	1.76	1.82

Abridged from Boyce and Evenson (1975), Table 2.7.

for granted "literacy, the roads, the implement factories, the banks, the marketing facilities, the commercial advertising, the programs for disease and pest control and the other facilities which in many countries are non-existent or inadequate" (1976, 132).

That a good deal more than just diffusion was required is illustrated by the change in understanding that Morss and his colleagues underwent during their multicountry study of small-farmer development projects. "We began our study on the assumption that the technology necessary for improved output and income for small farmers was available. . . . Instead we found that 61 percent (of available packages) were inadequate for one reason or another" (1976, 1:103). Jon Moris makes a similar point after extended experience in East Africa: "Take away improved on-farm water management and the associated movement to double and triple cropping and High-Yielding Varieties lose much of their attractiveness. . . . The alleged yield superiority of 'improved' technologies often vanishes when one introduces realistic labour, risk and input availability constraints into the evaluation" (1983, 3).

Technology developed for a particular microclimate and for particular credit, supply, and marketing characteristics may not produce a similar profit if applied elsewhere. Assuring that recommended technologies are appropriate (that is, that they are feasible for local farmers given available resources, and that they will produce a sufficient rate of return at an acceptable level of risk) has been a problem noted by most of the sources we have reviewed.

The failure to develop appropriate recommendations can be seen as the result of any or all of three causes. Only one is a failure of the information system. First, countries simply may not have the financial resources to undertake the extensive localized research that is most often recommended. Money, however, may not be the only issue; Evenson and Kislev (1975) show that the rapid growth of resources devoted to extension is not matched by new resources devoted to research. Shortage of talent and shortage of financing may both be problems.

There may also be no short-term research solutions to the problems of some environments. A small amount of local adaptation research may not be enough without other changes in the environment. Corn growers in rain-fed zones, with minimum access to credit and at some distance from input and sales markets, may not be helped much by even good short-term research. Without the complementary elements of Mosher's Progressive Rural Structure, it may not be possible to recommend any appropriate technology.

Our final explanation for the failure of research to produce appropriate recommendations is the poor integration of research and extension institutions. Extension field staffs are often unable to let researchers know what research is appropriate. Almost every source examined decried the inadequacy of links between farmers and research agencies. Rice argues that this was the result of a deliberate policy of United States advisers, at least in Latin America, who tended to "underrate the importance to the extension mission of functional linkages with other institutions" (1974, 417). Whether this was the case or the failure is endemic to all government bureaucracies is an open question. However, the tendency for government agencies to arrange top-down communication more efficiently than bottom-up and to resist coordination with other agencies, especially if that implies some reduction in autonomy, is not restricted to extension agencies. While the support for extension autonomy among United States advisers may have had some influence, the failure to link with research agencies may have gone on regardless.

In looking for ways to link extension and research agencies and to maximize the effect of farmers' needs on the operation of the agricultural agencies that serve them, one must ask whether a proposed strategy provides the incentives to agents and to agencies to act in support of those goals. Sincere calls for extension agent-researcher coordination with no rewards for that coordination, or demands that agents act as communication channels to research agencies for their clientele with no rewards for time spent performing that function will not change the current situation.

Training and Support of Field Agents
In-service training is universally endorsed, but it seems to be minimally implemented. Mosher has argued logically that constant in-service training of extension workers is more important than pre-service technical training, because few agents have sufficiently expert backgrounds to serve without regular subject specialist support. Yet as Coombs and Ahmed point out, in-service training rarely meets this consensus ideal: "Judging from our evidence in several countries, in-service training for extension personnel is seriously neglected.... India's 60,000 Village Level Workers typically get this [two-month] training every six years. Many now working...have had no refresher training...since the Green Revolution got started, yet they are supposed to be agents for spreading it" (1974, 132). Rice's description of Latin American systems is no more optimistic on this point. There is "no in-service training to speak of" (1974, 95). Moris describes the support for field agents in Africa in quite desperate terms. "The extension agent will be cut off from the flow of technical information, using as principal reference the tattered remnants of mimeographed notes from agricultural college days" (1983, 13).

Budget squeezes may reduce the support for this abstractly valued but de facto low-priority element. Typical in-service training, even if it were offered more widely, may also be unproductive. In-service training assumes that agent knowledge is dated, but if an extension system has no way of assuring that the research institution is producing appropriate new knowledge, then retraining is less relevant.

Long-term Efficacy
A very large number of small-scale agricultural development projects have started up since World War II. Often sponsored by foreign aid agencies and initiated with external technical staff, they may have received a positive appraisal at the end of their pilot phase, with a sober recommendation that they be expanded more broadly. More often than not, no expansion has taken place; if it has, it has fallen

far short of the expectations of the designers. Many explanations for the failure to pass beyond the pilot stage of development can be offered: the demand for talented people was beyond the local capacity to supply them, the demand for logistical support and organization was unreasonable when expanded beyond a local theater, expansion represented a threat to someone else's bureaucratic turf, or expansion demanded redistribution of scarce resources in favor of a politically weak constituency. Whatever the explanation, projects that cannot survive are unsuccessful projects. Institutional viability is often in doubt for innovative extension systems. Both Rice and Axinn and Thorat use the institution-building criteria developed by Milton Esman and his colleagues (Rice 1974, 85) to evaluate the strength of extension institutions.

The first criterion is sheer survival; and survival means establishing a call on the national budget. While it may be argued that the budgets for most extension services leave them poverty-stricken, the services are, if the evidence of Table 4.1 is to be accepted, able to survive and expand. This is the major contrast between the conventional extension systems and many of the innovative projects developed under postextension models.

Another criterion for evaluating institutional strength is the nature of the linkages that extension organizations maintain. We have already noted that, on this score, most conventional systems fare poorly. Crucial links with research institutions are said to be strained, and in many places agents are limited in their ability to assure that complementary services (credit, modern inputs) are available. However, while not downplaying the problem of institutional isolation, we might ask whether that isolation is not the factor that allows systems to survive in the first place.

Isolation means direct reporting lines, a limited task, and fewer disputes over bureaucratic turf. It may ease the process of surviving, while it reduces the possibility of success in achieving improved productivity. That survival and success may be at opposite ends of a catch-22 situation is a hypothesis worth considering. There is no doubt, however, that all projects for serving large numbers of people over a long period need to take explicit measures to assure their survival. That may mean organizing a constituency in order to make demands on the political system. It may require simplifying the operational structure to avoid imposing too many complex tasks on field agents. It may mean locating ways to serve required functions that do not require highly motivated people working enthusiastically year in and year out. It may require incentives to keep agent turnover limited. As we look at subsequent projects, their success or potential success in solving this last problem — survival over the long run — will be a crucial issue.

APPROACHES TO RESOLVING THE MAJOR ISSUES

We have identified four more-or-less unresolved obstacles to doing successful extension: reach, appropriate recommendations, training and support of field agents, the long-term efficacy. A variety of strategies has been proposed and (usually) implemented to resolve those difficulties. In the next section, these strategies are presented in an order that reflects the major extension problem each is trying to resolve. Several address more than one issue, but stressing particular aspects simplifies exposition.

Extending Audience Reach

Conventional extension systems, with their reliance on one-on-one contact between extension agent and individual farmer, cannot directly reach the mass of farmers. Typically, while agents may be available for every 500 farm families under the best of circumstances and one per several thousand families under usual circumstances, most agents work only with 50 to 100 families on a regular basis. The other farmers are expected to learn indirectly as they observe what directly served farmers do, or hear from them about new techniques. However, since the contact farmers are relatively advantaged and often have resources and problems different from those of most farmers, the trickle down of information is said to be unsatisfactory. Ascroft and Gleason (1980) describe the Kenyan diffusion system, which "consisted of an authoritarian top-down model which reached only the same already-converted, over-endowed farmers over and over again." How then does one reach the rest of the farming population? We organize proposed solutions in four categories: changing the contact farmers, multiple-tier strategies, learning centers, and organizing groups.

Changing the Contact Farmers. Some will argue that depending on natural diffusion — from farmers directly reached by agents to the rest of the population — is essentially a sound idea. If diffusion does not occur, the argument runs, it is in part because the wrong farmers have been chosen to be helped directly. Technology appropriate for elite farmers may be inappropriate for others, and in any case diffusion between elite and nonelite groups may be minimal. Opinion leader theory (Katz and Lazarsfeld 1955) requires that opinion leaders belong to the same social network as do those whom they influence; they are not members of an elite. Yet, if the descriptive literature is correct, it is the elite who are reached by the agents. If true opinion leaders can be found, the argument runs, and assuming that the offered technology is of value, extension that concentrates on those influentials will produce a multistep flow of information and innovations.

An interesting example of this strategy is the Kenya Tetu Extension Project, described in a series of reports by Ascroft, Roling, and colleagues (1973). Recognizing the progressive-farmer bias of most extension systems, the initiators of this pilot program developed a strategy to bring less-progressive farmers into agricultural training programs. They developed a progressiveness rating scheme (based on number of innovations adopted) and arranged for farmers who were less progressive than the average to participate in a three-day course, along with the Junior Agricultural Assistant (JAA) assigned to their zone. The course concentrated on the growing of hybrid maize for which an appropriate technology package was available. Farmers also received credit for all necessary inputs on a limited scale. When the farmers returned home and implemented the recommendations (and almost all of them did), they obtained continuing help from the JAA. The authors report that not only did course participants adopt the new technology but neighbors did also (an average of over twenty neighbors for each participant). This appears to be a successful attempt to extend the reach of the extension system by switching contact farmers. However, some caveats are in order.

It turned out to be difficult to recruit less-progressive farmers; only after repeated efforts were local extension agents and village leaders willing or able to arrange for other than the most progressive farmers to attend — and at best the farmers who attended were only a little less progressive than average. While it is reported that efforts to recruit less-advantaged farmers to extension programs, based on the Tetu model, have been expanded (Morss et al. 1976, 2:124), quantitative data are unavailable. It is worth noting that the collection of data for rating farmer progressiveness explicitly was abandoned by the third year of the project, to be replaced by subjective identification of participants by field agents.

Also, while the authors imply that diffusion is greater than it would have been if the more-progressive farmers had been the contact farmers, there are, in fact, no data comparing more- and less-progressive farmers as contact agents. It might be that the more-progressive farmers would have been even more successful as diffusers than were the less-progressive farmers.

Finally, the project represents special circumstances. Tetu is one of Kenya's most advanced areas. A very large percentage of the farmers who were reached had been visited by an extension agent in the previous year. There was an appropriate technological package ready for distribution; in many circumstances the major problem limiting diffusion from elite to nonelite farmers was the difference in technology appropriate for the two groups and not the lack of a communication link, which was the focus of this project. The project had the close attention of highly trained outsiders, including foreign advisors who were able to ease bureaucratic obstacles to the operation of the project. While such procedures are appropriate in the research and development phase of a project, they do not allow us to make easy generalizations about normal circumstances.

Multitier Strategies. When paid extension agents cannot reach a large enough number of farmers, some projects have recruited additional tiers of paraprofessionals. Each well-trained agent supervises a cadre of paraprofessionals who are responsible for most fact-to-face instruction. The paraprofessionals are locally recruited and serve as volunteers or are paid at a low rate. Because they are locally recruited they are more knowledgeable about local farmers' needs. If they farm their own land, they can use it for demonstrations.

One realization of this multitiered system took place in The Gambia in a World Bank–sponsored rice-growing project (Morss et al. 1976, vol. 2). Based on a technological strategy developed in a Taiwan-sponsored project, the project used paraprofessionals to work under agricultural extension agents as "demonstrators." Morss and his colleagues describe the paraprofessionals as follows: "They receive intensive training from the project for about a month and then each is assigned to work directly with the farmers. The demonstrator is paid by the project during the first crop cycle, after which the cooperative assumes responsibility....One government agricultural officer supervises the work of three demonstrators; monthly seminars are held for the demonstrators during which additional training is provided and operational problems are discussed" (1976, 26). The available documents provide only a preliminary evaluation, which describes large, cost-beneficial gains in production but does not specifically analyze the role of the demonstrators.

The Gambia project illustrates two important issues in the development of multitiered extension effects. To the extent that the paraprofessionals' skills are limited, their value lies in their fidelity as communication channels between client and extension agency. Without the level of continuous training that occurred in The Gambia, the paraprofessionals may become ineffective as time and distance attenuate their ability to serve as a communication channel. Also, The Gambia made use of a tightly designed strategy in which the role of the demonstrator was narrowly focused on a defined set of activities. Attempts to use paraprofessionals or volunteers in a less-structured way are not as likely to succeed.

In Guatemala, hundreds of volunteer community leaders were trained in six-week courses. Senegal's Animation Rurale and India's Community Development also trained local workers and, in addition, paid them. In all three cases, the trainees were to serve as catalysts of agricultural and other social change in their communities. There is some doubt that they did. The problem with this strategy is twofold. The low pay, or lack of it, must be set against the heavy demands for motivation and skill. The rewards consist largely of esteem and gratitude from those in the community, and perhaps easier access to outside resources. Whether such rewards are of sufficient magnitude to maintain the action of volunteers for a long time is in doubt. In addition, programs that are limited to training volunteers often stop there. Once the volunteers return to the community, where there is no structured educational program, the probability of its rapid disintegration is high. Even if volunteers are effective leaders, their own knowledge of agricultural practice may not surpass that of other farmers. Without regular input from outside, it may turn out that before very long the volunteers have little to offer beyond group-organizing skills. The rewards of participation for volunteers and for farmers will not be high.

The Learning Center. Some have argued that an emphasis on extension agents is misplaced; the goal is to provide information for which extension agents are but one mechanism. From this perspective, the primary effort must be to improve access to information. It is argued that if the information is useful and available in a comprehensible form, people will seek it out and learn a great deal on their own without complex delivery systems.

The *learning center*, to be filled with materials that enable individuals and groups to find what they want to know and to learn at an appropriate speed, is a logical outgrowth of this argument. No large-scale versions of such a system exist, and thus there is no evidence on which to judge its value. Its promise lies in its ability to provide material on a wide variety of topics, unlike extension services, which, of necessity, have a much narrower coverage. Also it leaves control over learning in the hands of the learners and not in those of distant and rigid central authorities. Finally, because it makes materials available locally, it can be used both by different people and by the same people returning for reinforcement.

There is another side, however. While it may be true that the best explanation for failure to learn is lack of opportunity, one cannot assume that, if there were the opportunity, learning would automatically follow. The history of self-teaching programs of whatever sort is not an optimistic one. Dropout rates are extremely high. The reliance of such programs on self-discipline, on returning day after day when the only reward is the value of what has been learned, has often doomed them.

A second and perhaps graver threat is the sheer administrative complexity of organizing enough of these centers to give the mass of farmers access to them. The prospect of preparing a large number of materials in a variety of media in locally appropriate versions, of distributing them to secure centers, and of maintaining the centers and their collections is an awesome one.

In sum, the learning centers' strength lies in their theoretical flexibility and local control; their weakness lies in their lack of learning structure and the administrative nightmare they might become.

Organizing Groups. Certainly the most commonly endorsed method for extending reach is the organization of local groups, where the effects of an extension agent can be multiplied. We have quoted previously from Milton Esman's argument; it is widely shared.

Groups — in the abstract, at least — can serve agricultural information in a variety of ways. In an obvious way they are cost-reducers, at least compared to one-on-one communication strategies. However, cost is not their primary advantage. They can also make understanding content easier. In a group, the right questions are more likely to be asked, the key objections raised. Also, if the content is developed at a central location, discussion by a group may provide an opportunity for localization of the message. A well-trained group leader can ensure a discussion of how a particular notion can be applied locally.

A group can also provide long-term motivation for continuity. When a program requires continuous attention to a curriculum over a long period, isolated individuals depending on self-motivation are likely to drop out. The learning process, often difficult and frustrating, must have its own rewards if any but the most strongly goal-oriented are to stay the course. The group meeting as a social event can provide such day-to-day rewards.

Also, a group provides social support for change. Individuals do not change their behavior in isolation. They live in integrated communities — the behavior of one individual is, in part, a reflection of the expected responses of his or her family and neighbors. Particularly when new behaviors represent substantial departures from community practices or norms, social support and encouragement are likely to ease change. This is particularly true of relatively powerless persons, like women in many rural societies, who are least able to challenge the status quo successfully as individuals. A person's willingness to change, particularly if it entails some risk, is likely to be magnified by the knowledge that others will change also.

The documentation on the role of groups in agricultural programs contains many examples of communal action: obtaining credit as each member becomes a guarantor of the loans taken out by others (Plan Puebla in Mexico is a widely known example), purchasing inputs or marketing surpluses as a cooperative, and farming land in common (as in the Agricultural Enterprise Promotion Program in Ecuador). There are, in contrast, few well-documented examples of programs (except for some media-using projects discussed in the next chapter) in which information diffusion occurs primarily in organized groups.

It is true that most extension agencies rely on group meetings for some educational purposes. But if the ECA-FAO study on African extension holds for other systems, that most often means group method or result demonstrations and only rarely group talks. And all group education is decidedly secondary to personal visits.

Taiwan's farm information system seems to be an exception to this pattern. Local farmers' associations hire extension agents (out of income from credit activities) who are affiliated with a broader research and extension service. Group meetings are the method of extension most frequently used by these agents, although farm and home visits are also common (Lionberger and Chang 1970). Axinn and Thorat describe the meetings as follows:

> The farm study . . . groups meet in the evening, once every two weeks (or at least once a month) either in a member's home or in a public place, such as a village temple. The group usually has about twenty members and its meetings also are attended by the . . . extension agent. . . . Study groups involving men [include] . . . groups dealing with land improvement, fertilizer uses, and varying kinds of cash crops, called special study groups, or commodity study groups if they focus on a particular cash crop. . . . At the study group meetings which are completely voluntary, the farmers exchange information on their own farming experiences and the extension agent in attendance gives new information (1972, 79).

The available information does not permit any direct evaluation of the success of these Taiwanese groups. However, they do form part of a research and extension system that is linked to a highly successful transition from traditional to modern agricultural practice.

Farmers' training centers are a final method of extending reach, since they bring groups of farmers together for one-day to several-month training courses. For the longer courses, however, the costs per farmer reached are high and the absolute number of farmers reached is quite small. In Malawi (Perraton et al.) a one-day course costs $4 per farmer and a five-day course $30, without including the cost to the farmer in time lost from farm activity. If they are simply a supplement to conventional extension, they typically exacerbate existing inequity of service, since participants are recruited from the farmers already being served by extension (Coombs and Ahmed 1974).

Appropriate Recommendations

Broadly speaking, there are two paths to assuring that a farm information system is supplying recommendations that are appropriate for farmers. Agricultural institutions can adapt the recommendations to fit a farmer's present environment, or they can attempt to change a farmer's environment to fit the recommendations. The first approach includes a variety of feedforward strategies to make a system responsive to farmers' needs. The second encompasses the widely endorsed integrated rural development strategies, in which agricultural information accompanies changes in credit, input supply, marketing, and perhaps other institutions that make it feasible to adopt recommended practices.

Feedforward Strategies. Agricultural research and extension institutions must do three types of investigation. First, through basic research on seeds (or other input factors), they develop an ideal variety for a particular ecology. Second, through adaptive research, they define complete technological packages adapted to given microclimates and social and economic environments. Finally, they develop information to respond to particular, often short-term, problems that surface during the crop cycle. Research resources, however, are limited. Institutions need to decide what resources are to be committed to the development of each type of knowledge, and then how to allocate the available resources within each area.

Do the basic research institutions concentrate on developing a seed ideal for commercially farmed rice grown on irrigated land, or do they develop a corn hybrid ideal for subsistence farmers in rain-fed highlands? Or do they minimize basic research and concentrate on adapting seeds generated elsewhere for similar ecologies? At the level of adaptive research, for whom is the package to be developed — the subsistence farmer with little access to credit, or the commercial farmer who has access to a tractor? Finally, what resources are to be devoted to answering the subsistence farmer's questions about the blight affecting his beans, and what to answering the commercial farmer's questions about the ideal time to spray insecticide on his cotton crop? Part of the answer to these allocation questions is political: who gets what scarce resources depends on who has the power to demand what. Part of the answer is technical: what a given research agency can accomplish depends on its talent pool. But part of the answer may be informational: whose needs are communicated to the research institutions? We shall ignore the obvious point, that allocation of access to the information system is a political decision, and concentrate on alternative mechanisms for giving access, assuming that there is a commitment to making the information system work better for now-unserved farmers.

Insofar as we have found, little explicit effort has been made to make basic research responsive to a formal feedforward mechanism from farmers. While basic researchers have certainly had to be aware of farmers' problems, the relatively long development time of this work and the isolation of research institutes has meant that feedforward has been indirect and informal. As Lionberger and Chang describe the Taiwan farm information system: in contrast to the systematic information links of lower-level research agencies, the agricultural colleges, which seem to do much of the basic research, have only haphazard contacts with extension workers and farmers.

We turn immediately to the next level of research, adapting the available products of basic research to local ecologies, generally in the form of recommended technological packages. There are four feedforward strategies (sometimes used complementarily) that we find repeatedly in the literature: experimental strategies, participation strategies, baseline investigation strategies, and farming systems approaches.

Most extension services use method-and-result demonstrations on exemplary village plots as a primary tool. Their purpose is to show farmers how much can be achieved with a new technological package. In some situations the results have been less than expected. Often the farmers who adopted the recommendations have done less well than has the extension agent who cultivated the demonstration plot (Morss et al. 1976).

The *experimental strategy* adds a step to this process, allowing farmers to try out the technological package; the package is then modified in response to farmer reaction. The Northern Cauca project of the Colombian Agricultural Institute illustrates the process of experimentation (Morss et al. 1976, 2:315). The extension system supplemented its usual activities by recruiting volunteer farmers to make comparative tests of newly developed crop varieties and traditional strains. They provided all inputs and allowed farmers to keep the harvest. When a test proved successful, a field day was organized for other farmers to view the results. In this project (which also helped arrange for credit and did additional extension education through organized groups), a reasonable proportion of target farmers adopted the recommendations and achieved yields commensurate with those on demonstration plots. Unfortunately, prices for crops declined in response to an oversupply so that even with increased yields, farmers barely broke even. Morss and his colleagues attribute this to the failure of the project organizers to consider marketing activities. Many farmers deserted the project the next year, and indeed the project staff seemed to lose heart and conducted many fewer experimental trials during the following year.

Participation strategies bring farmers into the process of adaptation more directly. The legitimation of the farmers as sources of information about their own environment came only slowly to extensionists. As Coombs and Ahmed mention, "another widespread characteristic [is the] expert's view of the farmer — especially the small traditional farmer — as a simple, ignorant fellow who does not know his own best interests and has to be treated like a child" (1974, 126). They contrast this conventional extension view with that of self-help community development projects, which assume that rural people are competent to analyze their own needs and solve their own problems. Unfortunately, none of our sources gives a very full description of how, through participatory approaches, farmers are able to influence the shape of the technological packages that are eventually introduced. Morss and his associates give some examples of de facto rejection of approaches to making ancillary services (like credit) available. For example, in the Bolivian potato production project, local peasant organizations preferred the more conventional credit system to a sharecropping system. Lionberger and Chang's description of the Taiwan system includes research technicians' self-reports of the influence of the farmers: up to 60 percent report at least some role for farmers as sources of research ideas. We did not find any descriptions in the self-help projects that told how specific elements of the technological packages themselves were changed at the behest of local organizations.

Baseline investigation strategies bring social science to bear in defining how technological packages are to be introduced into a community. Before developing a package, project directors ask social scientists (drawn from agricultural economics, anthropology, and sociology) to examine the aspects of culture, existing agricultural practices, and institutional structures that are likely to affect the optimum shape of a technological package. In the Nigerian Uboma development project, nine months of intensive interviewing concerning physical environment, social organization, diet and health, land tenure, and agricultural practice preceded the definition of the project. Morss and his colleagues describe the results of this survey enthusiastically:

> The [research]...gave...a basic understanding of the problems facing [farm families], as well as ideas of specific innovations which could be imitated rapidly with tangible results.... A farming calendar was developed, with specific roles for men and women. The timing of agricultural assistance efforts was planned.... The family interrelationships were plotted...so the "natural" groupings of people could be used as means for launching various schemes.... This and other information was collected to determine the best means for building local involvement (1976, 2:238).

While such baseline surveys are in theory quite helpful — and apparently in this program they were so in fact — this is not always the case. The requirement for baseline surveys has become more widespread than the capacity to make use of the data gathered. Unless such research work is responsive to the decisions that a project is to make, it is not likely to be helpful.

A conceptually related but far more elaborate version of this strategy is currently being implemented in a number of sites in Nepal and Swaziland under the title *farming systems approach*. It involves the development of a sophisticated understanding of the opportunities and constraints set by the ecological and socioeconomic interrelationships in a farming environment. This leads to the specification of recommended changes not only in the technological package but in other elements of the agricultural structure. It starts with investigation and thus represents an example of a feedforward strategy for defining appropriate technology. However, the likelihood of its recommending systemic change makes it also an example of the next broad strategy for developing appropriate recommendations: integrated rural development.

Adapting the Farmer's Environment: Integrated Rural Development Strategies. There are some situations in which additional knowledge about appropriate recommendations will not lead to an adjustment in the package an extension system recommends. Such investigation may lead to the conclusion that no package will enable farmers to increase their earnings without concomitant changes in other rural institutions such as credit services, input supplies, and marketing systems. That conclusion, one that many sources suggest has become a consensus (if Coombs and Ahmed are correct), has led to *integrated rural development projects*. These programs assume that offering appropriate recommendations is not only a matter of locating packages that will do best in the current environment. Often, it is argued, increased productivity and profit will come only when improvements in the resource base match improvements in available information.

In Plan Puebla, for example, project sponsors did not merely develop and adapt a large number of locally appropriate technological pacakages. They stimulated the development of credit associations, arranged for extension services, expedited delivery of supplies, and took advantage of existing government price supports for corn (Morss et al. 1976, vol. 2). In the Kenyan Tea Development Authority project, the complex set of practices associated with tea growing was successfully introduced to about 80,000 small holders cultivating one-acre plots. The Tea Development Authority raises and provides credit, trains growers, defines completely appropriate packages, delivers supplies, closely supervises and inspects plant and leaf growth (one agricultural agent per 100 tea farmers), collects tea leaves for transportation to factories, and purchases tea at fixed prices.

The Puebla and KTDA projects no longer depended on adjusting technology to a constant environment (throwing information at a problem — a theme that resounds often in this book) but changed the environment to make it possible for consumers of information to make productive use of it. It is interesting to note that in the case of Plan Puebla, the participation of farmers fell short of what was hoped. Benito (1976) suggests that even a package as well tested and comprehensive as that offered by Puebla did not fit perfectly into the local environment. Many farmers apparently felt that the additional labor demanded by the recommended package took too much away from alternative employment opportunities and preferred not to participate.

Training and Support of Field Agents

That extension agents need constant retraining and technical support is widely acknowledged. That very few national extension services provide an adequate level of in-service training is also acknowledged. At best, along with irregular formal training opportunities, most systems provide some back-up subject specialists who are available to respond to questions raised by agents. Most systems de facto assume that agents can act autonomously: that they have the technical skills to help farmers analyze their problems, to suggest solutions, and to help farmers realize those solutions.

Moris claims that such an assumption is unreasonable; governments appoint "half-trained 'village workers' with from six to eighteen months of mostly classroom instruction. The technical issues that will arise probably necessitate a minimum of about three years solid scientific training. . . . The few staff with degree-level backgrounds are tied up . . . trying to keep the support system in operation" (1983, 13).

One solution to this problem is embodied in the World Bank's Training and Visit System, developed by Daniel Benor and described by Benor and James Harrison. It resembles Taiwan's farm information system (Lionberger and Chang) and particularly the highly structured development programs of the Kenyan Tea Development Authority and the tobacco plan of the Nigerian Tobacco Company (Morss, et al. 1976, vol. 2). However, the Training and Visit System is better known than these programs; and because it can be argued that it has attacked less tractable problems, we shall examine it with some care.

Its authors attribute extraordinary increases in yields in many crops (including cotton, paddy, and wheat) to the operation of the system in regions of Turkey and India. In many aspects it is similar to conventional extension systems; it relies on extension agents reaching contact farmers who are to serve as diffusion nodes for the 90 percent of the farmers not directly reached. The contact farmers are taught in more or less conventional ways. The extension agents do not supply inputs but serve as links between farmers and input suppliers.

What is sharply different in this system is its organization: its rigid structure and demand for extensive information flows among the several actors in the system. The Village Extension Worker (VEW) works on an explicit two-week schedule. One day every two weeks, all the VEWs meet with subject-matter specialists who train them in the tasks they will undertake during the ensuing two weeks.

> Efforts are concentrated, [only] three or four crucial points are covered. . . . One-third of the time [is spent] on the lectures . . . the remainder on practical field demonstrations of what is taught and on discussions. The VEW should be required to restate the lessons as he would present them to the farmers . . . [and] be given pamphlets summarizing recommendations as well as samples or other visual aids as required. The goal is to make the VEW a Subject Matter Specialist on the few points of particular relevance in the coming fortnight (Benor and Harrison 1977, 23).

The VEWs also have a second day of training each fortnight with their immediate supervisor "during which points raised in the previous week's training system will be reinforced" (p. 23). Both sessions offer VEWs an opportunity to raise problems they are having with farmers in the field. The rest of the VEWs' time is spent working with small groups of contact farmers, so that every group is seen once every two weeks.

Unfortunately, we have no independent evaluation of how the system works in practice, only Benor and Harrison's description of the ideal model. However, since that description is the product of many years' experience, one must assume that it represents the authors' view of what has turned out to be feasible. The authors admit, though, that "without dedication and particularly the enthusiasm which initially depends very much on the inspiration of the key personnel selected to put the system in operation, one might question whether it can be expected to succeed" (p. viii). More work is demanded of agents and their supervisors than in the conventional system. Nonetheless, Benor and Harrison argue that the success agents will have and the enhanced respect they will receive from farmers will generate the motivation to keep them working. Only long-term evaluation will indicate whether they are right.

One recent evaluation of a two-year-old Training and Visit System in Haryana, India, suggested that the operational model fits the ideal model in at least some aspects. Feder and Slade (1985) note that 60 to 70 percent of contact farmers report meeting with extension agents as the model suggests they should — once every two weeks. These authors also suggest that contact farmers are somewhat better off and of higher status than noncontact farmers, as is typical in extension systems. However, the expectation that noncontact farmers will also gain some benefit from the Training and Visit System was upheld. Between 20 and 50 percent of the noncontact farmers had at least one contact with the extension system in the previous month. This contrasts with only 11 percent of farmers who had extension contact in a neighboring state without the Training and Visit System.

Two additional comments about the Training and Visit System are appropriate here, although they do not bear directly on in-service training. First, the system requires a large number of extension workers, one per 500 to 1,000 families, and a dense hierarchy of supervisors and subject-matter specialists supporting them. While Benor argues that the returns outweigh the costs, many governments may be unwilling to bear the absolute costs of the expanded system. And in some places (Moris argues that East Africa is problematic in this regard), middle management, so crucial to this model, may simply be unavailable.

Second, Benor and Harrison (1977) argue that in the early stages of project implementation it will be possible to improve farming practices without demanding additional cash outlays from farmers. They argue that enough additional income and confidence will result from such no-cost recommendations that farmers will be prepared to invest in new inputs. Benor and Harrison are the only major source encountered that argues that information alone is enough to change farmer income. And one would expect that the extraordinary increases in yields they describe for Turkey and India, and which they attribute to the system, could not have been achieved without significant additional purchases of fertilizer. Clearly, their formulation, which assumes that significant improvements can result from the reorganization of existing resources, is radically out of step with most current thinking. It suggests a promise of substantial returns on investments in information flows; evidence to support this contention would be eye opening.

Long-term Survival

Two strategies are often recommended to ensure long-term project survival: participation and power. *Participation* does not mean that clients merely have some say in the operation of a system. It means that farmers are getting sufficient benefit from a system that they are willing to pay for its operation out of their (enhanced) agricultural income. In Taiwan, extension agents are partly paid for by cooperative income; in Nigeria the Tiv Bams (farmer's associations) fund their own credit operations and an extension service through savings and dues at the village level. In both cases, because the farmers are paying for the system, they can make sure it is responsive to their needs; and because the system depends on farmers' voluntary contributions, it has strong incentives to keep the farmers satisfied. The possibility for long-term survival is enhanced because the sponsors receive the benefits, and the incentives for eliminating unproductive activities are strong. In a government-sponsored or other third-party system, incentives for responding to farmer needs may be much less. However, the organization of such associations depends on strong communal cooperation; among both the Tiv in Nigeria and the Taiwanese, mutual financial support and cooperation has a long history. Other self-supporting farmers' associations have had varying success (Morss et al. 1976; Coombs and Ahmed 1974).

The second strategy is the development of political power. This is the strategy that some observers would argue accounts for the long-term survival of the United States extension services. If a farming constituency organizes its political strength so that it can successfully demand subsidies from a central government for its research agencies and extension activities, then that system has a reasonable chance to survive. However successful that strategy has been in the United States, the competition for scarce resources has come out less well for poor farmers in developing countries. Indeed some would argue that even in the United States, poorer farmers have been less well served by the extension service than have been better-off farmers (Rogers, Eveland and Bean 1976). In any case, successful recipes for enhancing political power are scarce, although many argue for the value of peasant organizations in developing such powers (see White [1977] for an example of such an effort in Honduras).

Another issue, which may not threaten long-term survival but does threaten long-term efficacy, is a high turnover rate of extension agents. Clearly if agents are constantly leaving the extension system, the possibility of maintaining an effective system is reduced. It is likely that short-term agents are less able to build trusting relationships with farmers and are less knowledgeable about those farmers' needs.

There is little explicit consideration of methods to reduce agent turnover in the descriptive literature. Increasing salaries to be competitive is one solution, but one not likely to be implemented. Another would be recruiting field workers whose training does not make them attractive to private employers. Korea's move from college-trained to secondary-school-trained extension agents can be seen as an example of that strategy. Of course, less well-trained agents require a more structured backup system of in-service training and field supervision.

Another strategy is to reduce the isolation and frustration of extension work. Increased contact with the next level of supervision and backup may reduce the agent's sense of isolation. One suspects that the Taiwanese extension agents, who are closely linked with improvement stations, are less likely to be looking for ways out of the system than are the Latin American extension agents described by Rice, who may have a greater sense of being left dangling. Similarly, if extension agents are relatively successful at what they do, are highly regarded by the farmers they work with, and are rewarded by the agencies that employ them, they are more likely to stay with a system. The logic of this seems strong, but neither the isolation-versus-contact nor the frustration-versus-success hypotheses have empirical evidence. It is worth noting that, although Rice decried most extension systems as achieving little, his several surveys of farmers, of professional workers, and of people studying extension gave reasonably positive assessments of extension agents' work. The assumption that agents are highly unhappy with their work and have poor self-images may be incorrect.

Chapter Five

Communication Technology for Agriculture

Radio and other mass media have been used to support agriculture in many places. Axinn and Thorat called it "the most dynamic channel in the whole field of extension education in the decade of 1960s" (1972, 183). Hyman, Levine, and Wright (1967) surveyed experts who had worked on agricultural projects in less-developed countries and found that half had been involved in projects that incorporated mass media. Most case descriptions of extension efforts (see Morss et al. 1976; Rice 1979; Axinn and Thorat 1972) list radio and printed publications among the teaching methods employed. Nonetheless, most such uses of mass media are relatively minor, at least from the perspective of system managers and budgeters. They are not believed to play a central role in agricultural education. Daniel Benor has stated, "I do know that the media will have little impact unless their use is combined with an extension service. Farmers may listen but they won't follow" ("Interview...," 1978, 8).

In this chapter we shall examine that assumption. We look first at the ways media have been typically used; we then turn to projects that have used media in more central ways, like radio farm forums, radio schools, and feedback-based open-broadcast programs. We look for evidence that belies the "little impact" assumption in cases where evaluations have been done. We then turn back to our earlier typologies of information flows relevant to agriculture and the typical problems of extension programs and speculate about the potential of communication technology in these areas.

TYPICAL USES OF COMMUNICATION TECHNOLOGY

The radio farm program is, as we have said, widely available. The descriptive literature, however, is thin with regard to the details of how such systems function. Pieces of information about such programs exist in scattered sources, and from them we have assembled a composite that we hope is representative.

In 1974, Radio Nepal broadcast four fifteen-minute agricultural programs each week. They were produced by the Ministry of Agriculture in its Kathmandu office with a staff of three persons (Mayo et al. 1975). Done by a talented producer, they were designed to provide helpful agricultural information generally consistent with the current programs of the ministry. According to a radio-listener survey, the program called "The Old Woman and the JTA [Junior Technical Assistant]" was among the country's most popular. The cost per program (in the range of $15 per fifteen minutes of production) was very low, owing partly to Nepal's low salary levels and partly to a shoestring production operation.

This program was similar to those carried out in other small countries and in autonomous regions of larger countries. In Nigeria, a daily farmer's program, "Agbe Onije Amodun," was broadcast in the state of Oyo and elsewhere (Patel and Ekpere 1978). Twenty-seven local districts in India carried regular farm broadcasts produced by Farm and Home Cells of All-India Radio. In 1971 over 3,000 programs were broadcast (Mathur 1972). The Ministry of Agriculture in Afganistan contributed a twenty-minute daily segment to a longer program called "Village, Home, and Agriculture" with a staff of seven broadcasters working in two languages. Only one of the seven had academic training in agriculture (Stockley 1977). The ECA-FAO report (1971) on extension in Africa states that radio was used at every site studied by the project, including Ethiopia, Kenya, Madagascar (Malagasy Republic), Malawi, Senegal, Tanzania, Uganda, and Zambia. The Extension Aids Branch in Malaysia broadcast thirteen programs and was on the air for more than four hours a week. In Uganda agricultural programming was broadcast seven hours per week in nineteen languages (Nelson and Kazungu 1973). Lionberger and Chang (1970) cited agricultural programming in Taiwan, and Coombs and Ahmed (1974) mentioned agricultural radio as an activity of Korea's Office of Rural Development. Many more examples could be cited. However, the mere existence of such services says little about their value. We want to learn who listens, how relevant the material is to their needs, and what effects the broadcasts have.

Evidence About Listening and Effects

Where there is data, the evidence about listenership is quite positive. Rural people in Nepal who owned radios (only about one in 100 did) were likely to listen to the farm program. In western Nigeria, Kidd (1968) found that 40 percent of a sample (which included owners and nonowners of radios) preferred agricultural programs above all others. A later survey (Patel and Ekpere 1978) in the Oyo state reported that every person surveyed (of whom only half owned radios) listened to the agricultural programs occasionally and 83 percent listened frequently. Because the sampling plan was not described, the representativeness of these respondents is not known. Perraton and associates reported that, conservatively, 30 percent of farm families in Malawi listened regularly to agricultural radio, three times the number of families reached by the conventional extension system.

Whenever the issue has been investigated, there is evidence that farmers attend to agricultural radio broadcasts if they own a radio or can listen to others' radios. This may be seen as a contrast to the assumption that farmers have to be cajoled into listening by the sweet context of general entertainment programming. It appears, although the data are sketchy, that farmers are an easy audience to reach if they have access to radios. But then one must ask, if they are reached, are they affected? While some studies have examined this question, they have made use of relatively weak methodologies.

Two approaches are common: self-reports by farmers of whether mass media are the source of knowledge about a particular innovation, and the correlation of exposure to radio programming with adoption of innovations. Rogers and Shoemaker (1971) aggregated the self-report data for developing countries from five studies and suggested that mass media (printed materials as well as radio) represented first sources of knowledge about studied innovations for 30 percent of the respondents. Of course, the extent of such use of media was sharply conditioned by the availability of agriculturally relevant content.

Several studies directly examined the role of radio in places where agricultural radio was known to be available. Kidd (1968) found that 57 percent of his Nigerian sample listened to agricultural radio. These included 17 percent who told someone else about what they had heard and 23 percent (or 40 percent of the listeners) who reported that they had improved their agricultural practice as the result of listening to the radio. Between 2 percent and 16 percent reported radio as their first source of knowledge about eight different innovative practices.

In the Indian Institute of Mass Communication (1968) study of agricultural information flows, 13 percent of the farmer sample reported hearing first or second about high-yielding varieties from radio. Patel and Ekpere (1978) reported for their sample of Nigerian farmers that radio was more frequently cited as a source of information about chemical sprayers, fertilizers, and pesticides for cocoa than was any other printed or interpersonal source. For other innovations it was less frequently used.

Self-report data are difficult to evaluate. The particular circumstances of an interview may encourage one answer rather than another; farmers may not know or may be unable to articulate the sources of knowledge and influence on a particular behavior. The common wisdom (Rogers and Shoemaker 1971) is that media are at best minor sources of agricultural information, and then only at the first stages of the adoption process. However, since that generalization is based entirely on self-reports and reflects data gathered in countries with widely varying availability of agricultural media, we need not accept it unquestioningly. In particular, we need not accept its possible corollary that if agricultural radio alone is added to a situation, there may be increased knowledge but no increased adoption.

Correlational studies have begun to test this hypothesis, but they too fall short. Patel and Ekpere found that listening to agricultural radio broadcasts was associated with knowledge of agricultural practice. This relationship holds when controls for education and age are entered, but it is still possible that a causal inference from this result would be spurious.

The Indian Institute of Mass Communication found that in zones served by special farm radio programming, people were 20 percent more likely to report radio as their source of information about high-yielding varieties (HYVs) than people in areas with less farm radio. There was also some tendency for farmers in the special radio areas to report greater adoption of HYVs (63 percent versus 53 percent self-reported adoption). Unfortunately, while these data are consistent with an adoption effect of radio listening, it appears that the intensification of farm radio broadcasts was but one of a series of changes, including enhanced extension activity, going on in the special radio zones, so causal attribution is problematic.

David Kidd's Nigerian data (1968) showed a strong correlation between media exposure (which incorporated exposure to agricultural radio broadcasts) and both farmer knowledge (.39) and adoption (.32). While the relationship is somewhat reduced when controls for extension-agent contact and wealth of farmers are introduced, it remains significant at around .20.

Many other studies (Rogers and Svenning 1969; Contreras 1980) have examined the correlation between media exposure and innovation adoption and have usually found positive associations. However, these studies refer to general media exposure, not agricultural media exposure, and as such are not evidence about the role of agricultural communication.

The present data are intriguing and suggest the value of a careful study of the ongoing impact of regular agricultural radio programming. There is a great deal of it; when it is available farmers listen, and listeners appear to be more knowledgeable than nonlisteners and to adopt more readily. The data are now too thin to allow definite judgments about causation, but they by no means suggest that there are no effects at all. And, given cost considerations alone, radio is worth careful consideration. For Malawi, Perraton and associates estimate the cost per listener-hour for radio at $.004, about one five-thousandth the cost per farmer contact with an extension agent.

Major Problems of Typical Uses of Communication Technology

While the available evidence suggests that more exploration of the role of agricultural radio is worthwhile, the descriptions point to at least three widely shared problems of coordination that typical programs face. Consistently, there is mention of the difficulty of coordinating radio broadcasts with both the agricultural calendar in given regions and other ongoing activities of extension systems. There are several elements to this problem. In places like Nepal, where a national agricultural radio program serves farmers who are planting different crops in different climatic zones with different seasonal schedules, and with different technologies feasible, there is no hope of generating programs with very much specific advice for all farmers. In addition, broadcasting units in ministries of agriculture are often bureaucratically isolated from field agents and do not find coordination easy. Finally, program producers are generally isolated from the farmers they serve. They may have time only for preparing programs, and none at all to spend with audiences in the field. And broadcasting budgets rarely cover research for directly assessing farmers' changing needs and concerns (see Bammi 1983; McDowell et al. 1984).

This tendency toward isolation is exacerbated by the nature of media production. To casual listeners (or even to outside experts) fifteen-minute broadcasts, the physical products of the broadcast organization, may sound the same whether or not they are the result of intensive prior study of farmers' needs. Indeed, the effort that goes into assessing farmers' needs may reduce time spent for achieving aesthetic quality, and the well-researched program may play more roughly than the less well-researched one. However, the measure of success for educational broadcasting is not aesthetic quality but informational and behavioral impact — and that is likely to be profoundly affected by knowledge of the audience.

Agricultural broadcasters who are very isolated from farmers tend to become trapped. If isolation leaves them less able to produce useful programs, it also distances them from farmers' reactions. They are thus often guided by a misleading criterion of success, the program's artistic or technical quality. While this can be the result of a preference for isolation on the part of producers (whose expertise may not be in agriculture but in media production), it can also be the result of financial pressures within ministries. If a fifteen-minute tape can be produced with or without research, and no regular assessment of its effects on farmers is held up as a criterion of success, why pay for the field presence? Further isolation is the likely result.

IMPROVING THE UTILITY OF COMMUNICATION IN AGRICULTURE

Efforts to improve on the open-broadcast strategy have been focused in two directions:

1. making broadcast content reflect local contexts by decentralizing production and adding a link between farmers and producers; and
2. organizing listening clubs to support and localize the radio broadcasts, sometimes creating a link with extension agents.

In the following sections we shall describe some major projects that represent each of these directions. Some individual projects have gone in both directions, but we shall discuss them under the category in which their efforts have been most innovative.

Reducing the Isolation of Agricultural Broadcasters

"Village, Home, and Agriculture" (Afghanistan). Trevor Stockley (1977) describes a program of technical assistance to rural broadcasting in Afghanistan that had three aspects: the intensive training of producers, the effort to make sure that agricultural broadcasts correspond to farmers' needs, and the development of a cassette-tape information program. The second of these has turned out to be of most interest.

Over a two-month period in a particular region, sixteen meetings were held with 400 farmers and their local extension agents. "From these meetings a priority list of the information needs of our target audience was drawn up. This list was scored in terms of an ability to provide useful information on the subjects listed and on the ability of the farmers to implement. . .advice" (Stockley 1977, 4). Over the following six-month period, weekly broadcasts of the national farm programs were addressed to those needs. While the report did not describe the process of transformation from farmer comments to program content, the approach seemed both effective and economically feasible. Stockley did not mention whether the link with the field was maintained after the experimental year.

The evaluation of the project included before-and-after surveys with an apparently representative sample of the farming population. It focused on the creation of an awareness of the five topics addressed by the programs (control of rye grass in wheat, of rust in wheat, of smut in wheat, of mice, and pruning). Substantial increases in awareness were reported (12 percent beforehand and 40 percent afterward were aware of each of the topics, on average), with between 7 and 33 percent citing radio as their source of information about the items. Since extension agents (as well as the cassette recordings) were diffusing related information, the awareness due to radio was almost surely an underestimate of the effects to be realized if only radio had been available. Indeed, when Stockley considered only those people who had heard about an innovation during the experimental period, about half cited radio as a source. Sixty-five percent of all respondents described the radio service as a useful source of agricultural information, and 42 percent considered it the most useful. These answers may have represented some "be-nice-to-the-interviewer" responses. The interviewers' self-identification (as a member of the radio unit or not) was not mentioned.

Because only awareness (not comprehension or adoption) was surveyed, it is easy to read too much into these results. (Intention to try an innovation was measured, but agreement was virtually universal among those who were aware of the innovation.) The effects of the renovated radio broadcasts were difficult to separate from those of the simultaneous cassette and extension activities, and the possibility of bias lent by interviewer identification cannot be eliminated. Nonetheless, the popularity of the program seems real enough and the programs were perceived as useful. The use of feedback from farmers and extension agents in defining program content may represent a low-cost, but important, improvement in the typical isolated production service.

The Satellite Instructional Television Experiment (India). India used a borrowed satellite in the early 1970s, and tested it as a transmission mechanism for development programming — largely using television and reaching 2,400 villages over one year. About 12 percent of the broadcasts of the satellite instructional project year were dedicated to agricultural instruction, with broadcasts three times per week (Shingi and Mody 1976). Apparently, scripts were prepared by the Ministry of Agriculture and produced by SITE staff. There were both general agricultural programs produced for national telecasts and additional programs broadcast for subsets of the several regional sites.

From the descriptions (Agrawal 1978; Shingi and Mody 1976), the programs broadcast appear to be similar to those of conventional radio programs; regional programming was quite limited, and the process of assuring that programs were appropriate to farmers' needs depended on sometimes outdated Ministry of Agriculture sources. The evidence of the experiment's effect is limited to reports by resident anthropologists who noted adoptions credited to the broadcasts by a few farmers (Agrawal).

The major difference between this and conventional programs is the addition of a visual channel to an aural one. Given the mismatch between the centralized production of a new national TV network and the highly decentralized requirements of agricultural information, the project reveals the difficulty of using television in agriculture. Its "natural" centralized growth pattern in developing countries, given the high costs of production, is likely to limit significant regionalization in the short run. Whether this can be counterbalanced by the advantage of the ease of learning new methods from a visual source has not been tested. The ability to see how new techniques are implemented and observe actual growth in a demonstration plot seems to have more promise than merely hearing about techniques and improved growth on the radio. Nonetheless, if television is, for the foreseeable future, likely to remain a national medium in most countries and if agriculture in these countries is highly varied by microregion, television (even community television) can have only limited promise over the next decade.

Masagana 99 (Philippines). In 1973, the Philippines launched a massive national campaign to improve rice production. Within a few years, apparently as the result of the campaign, the country had switched from being a rice-importing to a rice-exporting nation. The program incorporated an explicit, research-based, sixteen-step strategy for improved yields; 3,200 new extension technicians; new programs for making available seeds, fertilizer, irrigation pumps, and credit; a system of price supports; and a very large mass-communication component. Eventually, 600,000 farmers were official program participants — although these had been reduced to 250,000 by 1978 (Academy for Educational Development, October 1978).

The mass communication campaign began with precampaign radio spots describing what the program was about and promising newly available credit. During each growing season, 125 radio stations broadcast a total of 50 daily local agricultural programs. The farmcaster on each program would inform farmers which of the sixteen steps they should be following at a given time, and also provide other useful information. The radio programs were supplemented by a widely distributed pamphlet that described the sixteen steps in detail. Other media were used to support the campaign also. The farmcasters, according to published reports (AED, October 1978), were not merely readers of copy supplied elsewhere.

The agricultural broadcasters involved in this project serve as more than disc jockeys. They act as information officers in the Provincial Action Committees,...answer queries from listeners, tape interviews with both information suppliers and information users, conduct research related to broadcasts, and attend community activities related to food production. In addition...[they] stay abreast of the informational and educational activities of all agricultural and rural development agencies.

The effects of the media campaign cannot be separated from those of other elements of the campaign — both those that provided incentives to increased production and those that were alternative information sources. Obviously the Philippine government had no interest in performing a cost-benefit experiment for the benefit of others who might want to replicate the program, but threw all resources into the fray in the quite reasonable hope that the chances for success were increased by doing as many different activities as possible. However, that leaves the observer with no way of defining the role of the farmcasters, whose links with ongoing local agricultural activity appear to be as strong as in any broadcast system we have seen described.

It is worth noting that the Philippine program operated under special conditions not always applicable elsewhere. For a very large number of rice farmers over much of the country, the appropriate recommendations were sufficiently similar to be defined in a sixteen-step procedure. This provided substantial opportunity for the standardization of much of what was to be broadcast, a major advantage for a media-based campaign. In addition, the Philippine farmers were often literate, and radio receivers were wide available. Pamphlets and daily radio broadcasts have special promise in such circumstances.

Basic Village Education (Guatemala). The Basic Village Education experiment (BVE) is probably the most conceptually complex, and is certainly the most intensively evaluated, program of agricultural radio directed to individual listeners we describe here. It began to operate in both Indian and Mestizo areas of Guatemala in 1974 and the evaluation activity was completed in 1977. It was presented in several versions (with radio broadcasts alone, radio supplemented by monitors, and by both monitors and an agronomist), but for this section we are most interested in the radio alone version.

USAID funded this program in order to discover how radio could optimally affect the pace of agricultural change. While the project was administered by the Guatemalan Ministry of Education, much of the control over the design and implementation of the project rested in the hands of foreign advisors (AED, September 1978).

BVE's most impressive characteristic was the major effort that was put into the preparation of radio programs. Extensive research preceded decisions on appropriate content; the design of the curriculum was an immensely careful operation and closely responsive to the agricultural cycle. Each day's "Agricultural Magazine," the culmination of this effort, was broadcast on the project's own transmitters.

Feedback mechanisms were judged to be indispensable to the success of the project. They included weekly feedback reports from monitors and field agronomists, testing of newly developed program materials, letters received from listeners (70,000 during the course of the project), listener surveys, and radio-signal penetration tests.

Although the evaluation of the program included comparisons among all the treatments, we shall focus on the effects of radio alone. The essential contrast is between random samples of subsistence farmers drawn from zones that received the radio signal and zones that received no signal in three distinct regions. The measure of success was before-and-after change on a thirteen-item scale of self-reported agricultural practices, including land preparation; seed choices; insecticide, herbicide, and fertilizer use; treatment of crop residues; storage practice; and credit use. The scale was defined by agronomists' notions of ideal practice, but individual items were not validated against productivity. Thus change on the practice scale may or may not have corresponded to productivity improvements.

Of the radio-versus-control comparisons in the three regions, one shows a significant and large gain in favor of a radio area (6.3 points versus 3.2 points on a 65-point scale), one shows slight advantage to the radio area (4.0 versus 3.2), and one shows no difference (1.01 versus 1.07). Each of these results represents data gathered after two years of project operation. Thus there is some (albeit inconsistent) evidence of a radio-broadcast-induced practice change.

Interpretation of the data, however, is problematic. Substantial preexisting differences existed between control and treatment zones, which may have meant different degrees of openness to change regardless of the availability of the educational broadcasts. In the region where there was no difference between treatment and control and little overall practice change, the radio signal spilled over considerably into the control area. That region also showed a relatively higher initial practice level, suggesting that there was some limit on just how much additional increase was possible. Both of these would suggest that the potential effects of radio were obscured by the evaluation design. Credit availability may have constrained just how far up the practice scale all farmers could go. The final report notes that credit access was a continuing problem (AED, September 1978). Farmers who might have responded to radio messages may not have because they could not afford the recommended practices.

A fundamental issue relates to the time span of effects and the sampling strategy. While two years may seem to be a sufficent amount of time to wait for widely diffused effects, it actually may not be enough. Since the process of radio-based diffusion is likely to begin with relatively few farmers who are ready to follow broadcast suggestions — suggestions that diffuse slowly as informal interpersonal channels reinforce broadcast ones — two years (and only two crop cycles) is probably too short a time to see maximum effect. Since the sampling strategy looked for effects among average farmers of the zone in which transmissions were available, such delayed diffusion effects were likely to have gone unmeasured.

On the other hand, we do not know whether the advantages in practice that were related to radio use have any implications for productivity. Other studies have shown that adoption of some recommended practices, in isolation from other changes, does not always lead to increased productivity (O'Sullivan 1980). It may be, for example, that increased use of fertilizer is not an important consequence of radio exposure and that only fertilizer use has important implications for crop yield.

There are some rough estimates of the costs of a potential expansion of the project to serve a zone of 100,000 farm families with a daily radio broadcast. Even incoporating the very high costs of technical assistance and evaluation related to foreign sponsorship and the experimental perspective, the cost per farm family is $2 to $4; without those costs, the annual expense per farm family would be $1 to $2 (Klees in AED, September 1978). (This excludes the cost of the farmer's time while listening to the programs.) It contrasts with an estimate of $35 to $63 for a traditional extension system per farm family.

The BVE project represents a major step forward in the realization of a radio-based agricultural information strategy. Its programming process is of great interest. Unfortunately the evaluation results remain substantially ambiguous, despite a great deal of effort, and leave us unable to judge its worth.

While broadcasts aimed at individual listeners are extremely common, only a few have been well described or evaluated. We shall synthesize what is known about their potential below, but first let us turn to the second major radio-based approach, that which links radio broadcasts to group activities.

Organizing Local Groups

Radio Farm Forums. Radio farm forums were founded during the late 1950s and early 1960s in a number of countries in Asia, Africa, and, in at least one case, Latin America. (These include India, Ghana, Iran, Zambia, and Costa Rica.) They involved the organization of groups of farmers who listened to a weekly or semiweekly broadcast and held a postbroadcast discussion of whatever topic was presented. Listening and discussion were expected to lead to either individual or communal action. After each week's broadcast and discussion, forum convenors were expected both to provide feedback to the central organization and to relay questions about unresolved substantive issues that would be discussed in a subsequent program.

There is relatively good evaluation of three early UNESCO-sponsored experimental radio forums in India (Mathur and Neurath 1959), Ghana (Coleman and Opoku 1968), and Costa Rica (Roy, Waisanen, and Rogers 1969). However, we suspect that these differ sharply from later nonexperimental expansion in those countries and elsewhere, and the descriptive data about the later forums is much less rich (Schramm et al. 1967; Klonglan 1967; Rundfunk und Fernseh and Africa Asian Bureau n.d.). We deal first with the experimental versions and then the expanded ones.

In all three experimental versions, a limited number of farm broadcasts (from ten weeks in India's Poona trial to fifty-two weeks in the Costa Rican experiment) were transmitted to a controlled set of village forums (4 in Costa Rica, 60 in Ghana, 145 in India). The Costa Rican project emphasized agricultural topics and attempted to correspond to the seasonal agricultural routine. The Indian and Ghanaian projects took a radically different approach; they chose twenty highly varied topics associated with development, with only a small proportion including specific agricultural recommendations. In both cases, decisions about appropriate topics were the result of consultation with all relevant constituencies, including development ministries and representatives of forum audiences. How much influence each constituency had on actual topic choice and script formulation is not described. The forums were organized by project staff recruited from sponsoring organizations. In both Ghana and India some forum participants were persuaded to attend because of their positions of authority and links with the government. While one suspects this kind of motivation will last through a twenty-week forum, it may not survive a longer period.

The evaluations of all three experiments are quite enthusiastic; there is reasonable empirical evidence of knowledge change in both India and Ghana; in Costa Rica the research results (albeit substantially in favor of forum villages) were plagued by problems of experimental mortality, preexisting differences between control and treatment groups, and an already dynamic agriculture, all of which make attribution of the cause of the observed differences problematic.

The forums, as they were organized, had three functions over and above those served by ordinary agricultural broadcasting: in both India and Ghana they extended radio's voice to more villagers since most participants did not have receivers. In all three countries they supplied opportunities to discuss communal issues with fellow villagers and come to joint solutions, or at least receive local reinforcement for a new practice. The forums also served as rich feedback channels to broadcasters to reduce their usual isolation.

However, although they served such functions successfully, they also indicated the difficulties longer-lived and expanded versions of such projects would face. Projects started in later years found that many potential participants already owned a receiver or were able to listen to their neighbor's. Communal listening, which entailed leaving home after a day's work, was no longer so attractive. It required consistent efforts at organization and a constant renewal of incentives for participation. In Costa Rica, the average attendance rates over the course of a year fell substantially, with the final average attendance reaching about half of the original total (Roy et al. 1969). Neither Ghanaian nor Indian evaluations report rates of change in attendance, but other radio study group campaigns have had a similar falloff in attendance after some weeks of operation (Hall and Dodds 1974).

Maintaining the operating radio forums turned out to be quite a difficult job. Within a year, more than half of the Poona forums had disbanded when the professional organizers were reassigned to other tasks (Schramm et al. 1967). And while as many as 12,000 forums were created in India subsequently, organization continued to be a major task, and many soon stopped operation. Even the 12,000 that had existed represented a 50 percent shortfall in planned forums. A state's success in organizing forums was related to the extent of its professional organizational activity. At their height, forums were available for perhaps 1 out of 15,000 people in the most successful states and 1 out of 100,000 people in the less successful states. Casual evaluation of the expanded programs also suggested that relatively better-off villagers were more likely to be involved, and that fewer than half of the registered members attended forums when they were held (Schramm et al.).

Organizational difficulties have also plagued the Indonesian radio listening clubs, formed with German technical assistance in the early 1970s. With 126 radio studios putting out 265 hours of rural programming, it was thought that greater advantage could be taken of broadcasts if listeners were organized into groups modeled on radio forums. While official estimates put club numbers at 11,500 in 1973, attempts to verify their existence found 5,500 on official lists and fewer still meeting with any frequency. (The evaluation study suggests an upper limit of 2,500 that regularly meet.) Government representatives in the villages were often found to play a central role. Rural field agents were charged with organizing the clubs. While some may have done so with enthusiasm, there is a sense in the evaluation report that club participation depended less on local motivation than on local compliance with government demands. (One can scarcely help speculating that, once the immediate stimulus disappears, so will the club.) The evaluation (RUF-AAB 1974) notes that many club members did their listening in their own homes or in the homes of friends. Almost all respondents reported listening to rural radio, but even in a survey that provided ample opportunity to say positive things about government programs, fewer than one-third reported that the radio programs were useful.

The failure to find programming useful leads to the third function of radio forums, which has proved difficult to implement over a longer time: an effective feedback loop between audience and broadcaster. In the early programs, there was a good deal of consultation among farmers, experts, and radio producers in choosing topics; and regular opportunities existed to obtain feedback from forum leaders who sent weekly reports and from participants' letters that could be read and answered over the air.

If the Indonesian program is an example, close links become hard to maintain when the projects reach a large scale. With few exceptions, rural programming is done by producers such that the "definition and selection of program content is not determined on the basis of what quality requires or what is preferred by the listeners but as a result of the material that happens to be available" (RUF-AAB 1974, 44). Feedback channels fall into disuse; "several months can elapse between a letter being received and an answer being broadcast and...the listening clubs are not informed beforehand that their question is going to be answered" (RUF-AAB 1974, 81). From the descriptive material in the evaluation report, it appears that the isolation of the broadcaster who addresses farm forums is not much less than that of the typical farm radio broadcaster described previously.

Our skepticism about the long-term viability of radio farm forums is admittedly based on thin evidence. It reflects a close took at the elements that underlie the apparent success of the experimental programs (novelty, the lack of individual radios, intensive organizational work to initiate and maintain forums, careful programming, and a central role for farmer feedback) and the difficulty of realizing those conditions over the long term and in a large-scale operation. Certainly a further look at the Indonesian radio listening clubs and such activities as still exist in India or in Africa may contradict this; but, until new evidence is available, a certain pessimism is justified about the major benefits resulting from the flow of agricultural information as embodied in radio farm forums.

Having expressed our skepticism about the farm forum tradition, let us now turn to a similar tradition, the Latin American radio schools, and challenge that skepticism. The founding radio school, ACPO (Popular Cultural Action) of Colombia, although subject to substantial outside criticism, has survived for over thirty years with a major presence in the countryside.

The Radio School Movement. ACPO is the first of the Latin American radio schools and remains the best-developed example of them. While its successor organizations have moved in other directions without obvious success — with the possible exception of the Honduran radio schools (White 1977) — ACPO is an institutional wonder. Started by a young priest in 1947, it employs 1,000 persons, maintains 20,000 volunteers in the field, and has enrolled between 100,000 and 200,000 students each year since 1960 in its listening and fundamental education courses (Brumberg 1975; Morgan et al. 1980). Brumberg estimated that about 5 percent of eligible rural Colombians were enrolled in an ACPO course in 1968. Many more listen to the daily entertainment and information broadcasts, including "Buenos Días," its most popular program. "Buenos Días" is directed to farm families for an hour and a half each morning and includes "news items of interest to agricultural audiences, . . . practical home and agricultural advice, [and] weather" (Brumberg 1975, 13).

ACPO publishes textbooks to accompany its courses, a rural newspaper, and a book series for rural families. It also annually sponsors and trains hundreds of leaders for its local programs. While ACPO is best known for its radio school courses, which feature what it calls "fundamental integral education" (a mix of primary school equivalency, development motivation, spirituality, and some relevant rural knowledge), we are concerned primarily with its agricultural training.

All of ACPO's programming, including agricultural materials, is centrally defined and produced. As a result, agricultural programming cannot be as responsive to the agricultural cycle or to variations in appropriate recommendations, given cropping patterns and microclimates, as an ideal agricultural information system would demand. ACPO's approach to agricultural improvement has been to choose certain basic themes ("use a compost pile," "apply fertilizer," "rotate crops," "do not slash and burn") and pound away at them in regular courses, articles in peasant newspapers, and books, as well as in regular radio programs. More recently, certain materials have been organized into two-month courses using daily fifteen-minute broadcasts; but one assumes these are restricted to topics (like raising pigs) for which a national prescription is feasible.

To some extent, ACPO's community leaders, who stimulate and oversee all ACPO activity, may be able to localize agricultural content, since part of their six-month training at ACPO's leadership institute involves learning agricultural techniques. However, much of the task of giving specific, locally relevant advice is carried out by other institutions.

Given the range of practices ACPO has chosen to influence, we may ask, How successful has it been? In a relatively informal study, Brumberg contrasted two villages, one having a heavy ACPO presence and one being only lightly served. Fifty-six percent of his respondents in the heavy-ACPO community reported recent increases in agricultural production versus only 34 percent in the light-ACPO community. Most striking was that 80 percent of the changers in the ACPO community named ACPO as a major influence for the increases in production.

Morgan and his colleagues (1980) at Florida State University did an extensive survey of rural families in ACPO's operating zones, looking at the association between exposure to ACPO and changes in agricultural practice. McDivitt (1981), using the Florida State data, examined the additional contribution of exposure to ACPO's agricultural programming, over and above the influence of background characteristics (education, economic status, age), to adoption of ACPO recommendations. She found that ACPO's contribution to self-reported adoption of a range of innovations was usually small but statistically significant (accounting for between 1 and 2 percent of the variance). It had the greatest effect on the use of compost piles.

While ACPO is only in small part an agricultural information program and is not an alternative to an extension system (something that both the Basic Village Education program and some farm forum versions might have claimed), it still has done remarkably well in the area of expansion and survival, which seems to be the downfall of many other programs. What explains its relative success? Certainly its use of multiple channels must play a role. Unlike the farm forums, if the ACPO meetings stop, there are still the radio programs, textbooks, and newspapers, all carrying related messages. However, it is widely acknowledged that no single influence has been more important than the active involvement of the Roman Catholic Church and, specifically, the parish priest (Morgan et al. 1980; Brumberg 1975). "His active participation has tended to result in the program's success at the local level whereas his lack of participation has usually meant less acceptance for the programs in the locality" (Brumberg 1975, 55). All of the other programs represent efforts mounted from outside, with an effort to stimulate local involvement, but the links from outside to inside were always tenuous. ACPO, with its dependence on the parish priest, began with a much stronger organizational link and was able to build on it.

Thus far we have considered general media-based agricultural information systems. However, extension was but one of the six information flows of interest. We turn now to the remaining five — education, feedforward, organization, training, and market information — but only briefly.

OTHER MEDIA-BASED INFORMATION SYSTEMS

Basic Education
This area is too large to incorporate in a chapter on agricultural information. Programs to provide basic education to adults out of school are found in almost every country and, in many, mass media are included. Some review of them can be found in Schramm (1977) and Jamison and McAnany (1978).

Feedforward
An important part of the description of the projects already presented has been a consideration of how they assure, or fail to assure, the appropriateness of recommendations. We have seen that, with the exception of the BVE project and the multifaceted Masagana 99 project, projects that depended on broadcasting alone often lost contact with the field; and that even farm forums, with their built-in talkback function, tended toward isolation. The logical mechanisms for maintaining current and constant information flow from the farmers to the radio producers are reasonably well known. They include formal and informal data gathering, farmers' advisory councils, feedback from field staff, and letters directly from clients. Yet the institutional pressures of daily production and the bureaucratic separation of production expertise and field experience work against all but slow and highly indirect information flows from farmer to broadcaster.

There has been but one media-based project, to our knowledge, whose primary purpose has been feedforward, the Radio Dissou program of Senegal. In this program, a letters-to-the-editor format was transferred to a broadcast medium (Cassirer 1977). Seventy percent of broadcast materials were expressions of viewpoints, complaints, and questions from rural audiences. The rest were responses by government agencies to those comments or the provision of useful information. It was reported that substantial modifications of government policy were the result of the large-scale use of this feedforward channel — in part because President Senghor overruled the attempts of directors of criticized government agencies to have Radio Dissou silenced.

There have been suggestions that two-way communication capacity, if it were available, would ease the institutionalization of the link between farm and studio. Eliminating the need for travel and reducing the time between request and response would lower some of the hurdles to success. We know of no project that has incorporated telephones or two-way radios in linking farmers to central institutions, although in some locations two-way radios have been used to supervise extension agents.

Organization

Many of the projects described previously combine local organization and mass media in achieving their own educational objectives. At least a few — among them, ACPO of Colombia — expect participation in radio-based communal organizations to result in a spillover participation effect. In the Brumberg evaluation of ACPO, citizens of communities where ACPO operated intensively were more likely to participate in other communal development groups than were citizens in communities of lesser ACPO activity. Less formal data on the Indian farm forums suggested that group activities extended beyond what was specifically recommended by the radio broadcasts. Thus, media used as a stimulus and focus for community organization has some history.

While less frequently linked to programs with extensive agricultural content, some media based programs have had a broader political purpose. Both the Movimento de Educacão de Base (MEB) of Brazil (Coombs and Ahmed 1974), which was the site in which Paulo Freire's "pedagogy of the oppressed" was developed, and the Acción Cultural Popular Hondureno (ACPH) (White 1977) were originally radio projects modeled on ACPO of Colombia. In both cases, the radio schools became the focus of a broader effort; each sought to raise participants' understanding of the political forces surrounding them and of the value of joint action to change opposing social and economic structures. Intensive group discussion, in the case of the MEB project, and local mobilization efforts of ACPH were to bring about a rural-based countervailing power movement. The MEB efforts were substantially curtailed by the Brazilian coup in 1964. According to Robert White, the ACPH was somewhat successful as an organizing base for a broader rural political movement (Concorde) that, at the time of his evaluation, was influencing some policies in Honduras. In both cases, the specific content of the radio-based educational system was a minor element. However, the attracting power of the radio schools provides an impetus to local organizing efforts.

Training

In contrast to teacher training, there are, to our knowledge, no media-based programs for in-service training of extension agents. However, some programs that use radio or television to reach farmers also believe part of their mission to be the training of extension agents. Klonglan's evaluation of the Malawi radio listening club programs makes this point. In this version of radio farm forums, extension agents were given radios and were asked to meet with two different groups on a weekly basis and listen with them to broadcast farm forum programs. As is usual in farm forums, this was to be followed with a postbroadcast discussion. Klonglan notes "some . . . officials also considered the extension field worker as a potential receiver for . . . broadcasts" (1967, 25).

India's Satellite Instructional Television Experiment programs directed at agriculture improvement were also said to have indirect training effects (Agrawal 1978). It can be assumed that similar benefits are a possible consequence of any such farmer-directed educational programs.

Using radio for the direct training of agents (or cassettes or high-frequency radio, when the cost of dedicating AM or shortwave frequencies to this purpose is too high) is also a feasible option. It is easy to imagine that some portion of Benor's Training and Visit System program of biweekly seminars could be supplemented by radio broadcasts. This would be so particularly in countries where the costs of aggregating a large enough number of agents in one place to be trained are high. Many systems have found that in-service training is among the first elements to be discarded or reduced when cost pressures increase (Coombs and Ahmed 1974). If the cost of providing such training can be reduced through use of radio, it may be that this element of a system, which all observers see as crucial, is more likely to be maintained.

It is also possible that two-way communication can improve the quality of supervision of agents, enable them to coordinate more efficiently with other institutions (credit agencies and input suppliers) that serve the farmer, and also decrease agents' sense of isolation in the field. The logic for offering benefits is strong, although until field trials occur it will be difficult to specify cost-effectiveness.

Market Information

Perhaps no use of mass media in agriculture is more common than the broadcast of market information. While evaluations, or even detailed descriptions, of just what is done are unavailable, it is known that agricultural radio programs provide market price and weather information on a regular basis. What is not known is who benefits from current broadcasts, and what benefit might be gained if they were more widely available. The base question is whether farmers receiving more or less market information than they do now would act differently. Market prices act as signals for farmers in two ways: they indicate how best to allocate lands among crops at planting time, and they suggest what profit will be earned if surplus harvests are shipped at a given time. Market price broadcasts (or a two-way communication capacity that allows farmers to obtain price information individually) are of value if:

1. Farmers do not have alternative sources of information that are accurate enough ("enough" here means that the farmer would have acted differently if he had known the actual price).
2. Farmers have the capacity to vary their actions; that is, they must have the economic resources to purchase alternative inputs, the technical knowledge to make full use of those inputs at planting time, storage facilities, and an income cushion that will enable them to wait for optimal times for sales of crops.
3. Farmers have not, as part of the arrangements for obtaining inputs, committed themselves to selling through a given intermediary or at a fixed price.

How often these three conditions obtain, we do not know. If they are

common, then investments in market price broadcasts, and even two-way communication capacity, may be justified. We do know, from anecdotal information
gathered in farm radio program evaluations, that price broadcasts are valued by
some. In Malawi, interviewees regularly suggested that they wanted information
about market prices of tobacco and ground nuts (the interviewees, however, were
commercially oriented farmers) (Klonglan 1967). Agrawal (1978) reports the
response of one woman who cited the satellite instructional television farm price
broadcasts as the source of her decision to deny her produce to the local trader and
sell it for a higher price at a nearby market.

Chapter Six

Summary and Implications: Agriculture

THE ROLES OF INFORMATION

We began with what seemed a simple question: Is enhanced investment in agricultural information (particularly in communication-technology-based information systems) worthwhile? The answer is complex and, in many ways, unresolved. In this concluding section we try to summarize and distill.

We divided information flows into six types: flows to the farmer (education, extension, market information, organization), flows to the extension agent (training and supervision), and a flow from the farmers to the agricultural extension institutions that serve them (feedforward). Evidence for the value of investment in formal systems for the enhancement of these information flows turns out to be weak or missing. The effects of education are the best evaluated. They vary with the speed with which new agricultural technology flows in the system: the greater the flow, the better the return to education. The evidence about extension education effects is uninspiring; studies point to associations between extension and productivity but do not encourage causal inference — particularly when it comes to linking costs of extension with productivity benefits. No firm evidence can be provided about the effects of other flows.

While we do not have quantitative evidence about the effects of public sector investments in information flows, we cannot assume there are no such effects. Failure to find positive evidence is unfortunate, but it is not the same as finding negative evidence. By and large, we have failed to find trustworthy evidence altogether. Even the harshest critics of conventional extension do not deny its potential utility; on the contrary, they argue that extension information programs would be valuable if only they were done right.

INFORMATION PROGRAMS WITHOUT COMMUNICATION TECHNOLOGY

Critiques of conventional extension suggest a consistent pattern of strengths and weaknesses and, as such, define the problems that reforms must face. Conventional extension's primary strength is its pervasiveness and longevity. Most countries have some sort of extension service and have maintained it over many years. In almost every country such services have established a place within the government organization chart and a call on the national budget. While institutional longevity is not the same as quality of service, it is a necessary condition of such service. Many other approaches, while on the surface more promising, do not last past early phases.

The weaknesses of conventional extension fall conveniently into three categories: failure to reach enough farmers, inability to develop appropriate recommendations for the farmers who are reached, poor training (particularly in-service) and insufficient management support of field agents, including weak links with other agricultural institutions (such as research, credit, and marketing). There is, of course, a wide range of implementations of conventional extension systems; nonetheless reviewers share a belief that these weaknesses are common. There have been many attempts to reformulate conventional extension in order to lessen these problems. We looked first at those solutions that did not use communication technology.

Strategies for resolving shortfalls in reaching farmers include making first contact with more typical, less-advantaged farmers, adding tiers to the extension system so that trained agents work through less well-paid (or volunteer) field workers, creating learning centers where farmers may obtain the information they need, and organizing local groups in order to multiply the effects of extension-agent contacts. As a set, while some successes have been reported, these solutions suffer most from organizational problems, particularly the inability of a government bureaucracy to nourish and motivate a vast army of distant local agents or groups.

Attempts to reform conventional extension systems to make it easier to supply recommendations appropriate to farmers' needs fall into two categories. On the one hand, some approaches take farmers' situations as they are and attempt to define the information that will be helpful: feedforward strategies, which expand farmers' leverage on the agricultural institutions that serve them; experimental strategies, which involve the intensive tesing of recommendations under realistic conditions; participation, or self-help, strategies, which legitimate farmers as sources of information about what is most useful in their own environment; and baseline investigation strategies.

Other approaches, in contrast, define optimum practice packages and then provide not only the recommendations but also the necessary resources. These integrated rural development strategies may couple delivery of information with credit sources, close supervision, and rearrangements of input supply and marketing.

The several strategies to improve the quality of recommendations offer promise, but there is little available evidence to suggest their efficacy. The integrated rural development approach has produced some notable successes (as well as some failures); but it is very expensive and requires an extraordinary organizational effort that is perhaps beyond the current capacity of some countries' agricultural institutions.

The lack of in-service training and continuing supervision and support of extension agents, despite formal rules in most systems requiring such activities, is virtually a constant. Generally it reflects inadequate budgets and results in agents with little helpful information to diffuse, high agent turnover, and low productivity. The solution — to do more supervision and training — is not novel, but faces strong counterpressures. One widely noted attempt to alleviate agent isolation, the World Bank's Training and Visit System, creates a rigidly structured program of links with a support service of supervisors and subject specialists. While no formal evaluation is available, anecdotal reports on a number of Asian projects have been enthusiastic.

INFORMATION PROGRAMS BASED ON COMMUNICATION TECHNOLOGY

Communication-technology-based information programs are widely used in most extension systems. By and large, however, such uses play but a minor part. In their typical role, agricultural radio programs are brief weekly (or even daily) broadcasts, in which a general agricultural topic is discussed. Sometimes market or weather information may be included. Usually the producers of such programs depend on information from ministries of agriculture and may even include verbatim reading of pamphlets. Rarely do producers have any direct feedback channel from farmers, nor are their activities closely allied with concurrent actions of the extension system or other institutions. These poor links suggest that the amount of directly useful information provided by such programs, especially the details of farming practice, may be minimal. Despite this, listenership surveys, when they are available, suggest that such broadcasts are highly popular — a point we return to below. Some intriguing, if ambiguous, data suggest that learning results from program exposure.

The majority of agricultural radio broadcasts are designed as minor enhancements to conventional extension services. There are some cases, however, where communication-technology-based strategies have been asked to play a central role. We divide these programs into two categories: the first includes those that depend on radio as a major channel but make substantial efforts to reduce the isolation of the broadcaster from the farmers and from other agricultural institutions. The second links radio broadcasts directly with group activities in the field.

In the first category, the most notable projects are Masagana 99 in the Philippines, which, as part of a successful multielement campaign to increase rice production, incorporated "farmcasting" as a major component; and the Basic Village Education experiment in Guatemala, which used radio broadcasts as its core extension device. In both cases, producers/broadcasters could depend on a strong, structurally integrated information link to the farmer audience. Masagana 99, because it utilized radio as but one element of its integrated campaign, does not permit direct attribution of productivity improvements to that element alone. BVE showed substantial effects on self-reported adoption of new farming practices in at least some of its comparisons. However, there was no evidence that productivity (or the farm practices most associated with productivity, like fertilizer use) was affected. Whether that failure reflected a too-short data-collection period, inadequacy of the supporting rural structure (like credit shortages or high fertilizer prices) to justify changed practices, or an intrinsic failure of the information program cannot be determined. Despite the tentative-ness of the evidence drawn from such efforts, they are ground-breaking projects.

The second category — radio programs linked to local group activities — offers two main traditions: the radio farm forums that were widely implemented in Asia and Africa, and the radio schools of Latin America. Radio farm forums organized farmers in particular villages to listen to and discuss weekly broadcasts directed at development concerns. Broadcasts usually incorporated answers to farmers' letters about problems they faced. The radio schools, depending on the organizing efforts of local leaders, created local cells for mutual support among learners. While much of the radio schools' effort has been directed toward literacy education, agricultural materials have also been presented. In at least one case, Popular Cultural Action of Colombia (ACPO), this included separate courses for farmers.

The evidence for direct effects of group-based programs is ambivalent. On the one hand, early farm forums, according to their evaluations, resulted in some knowledge change. While data about innovations adopted and about productivity are absent, that is not the main concern. What most farm forums have been unable to do is survive. Dropout rates for even short-term experiments have been high, and the disappearance of large numbers of forums in their entirety has occurred in every longer-term program that has been evaluated. Creating and maintaining group-based farm programs over more than a few months requires an extraordinary and continuing organizational effort that has been beyond the resources of most who have implemented the programs. While the ACPO radio school has had major success in maintaining itself and its local activities over thirty years, it is a sharp exception to the general experience. Its success is often attributed to the active participation of the parish priests, a resource not always available elsewhere.

Finally, we looked for projects that used communication technology to enhance other information flows. With the exception of basic education projects (for which reference is made to other documents), there was little to be found. Despite suggestions that communication technology might help in the supervision and support of extension agents, and that market and weather knowledge might be improved via both radio and two-way technology, there was little systematic description of such programs and no evaluation.

IMPLICATIONS

What, then, is to be concluded from the preceding survey? What role does communication technology have in improving agriculture? For a long time, basic references in communication for development held fast to the argument that a local group structure or, at the very least, face-to-face communication was a necessity in agricultural programs. Our review of the evidence provides no strong support for that contention.

Arguments in favor of combining face-to-face with mass media channels rely on three assumptions:

1. People will not listen to informational broadcasts if they are not stimulated by a group.
2. People must have material reexplained to them (or made locally relevant to them) by group leaders or extension agents.
3. People are reluctant adopters and require group adoption as a support.

Yet the evidence, tentative as it is, can make contrary assumptions equally tenable:

1. People listen avidly to agricultural broadcasts, even when they may be of poor quality. While many farmers do not have radios, listener surveys suggest that both owners and nonowners listen regularly to agricultural programs when they are available.
2. Radio broadcasts can give quite clear instruction if they spend enough time preparing their materials. In particular, the need for a local channel to clarify doubts and reexplain material can be substantially reduced if the radio broadcast zones are reasonably matched to agricultural microclimates and an extensive program of feedback is incorporated in the production process.
3. People are not reluctant; indeed, they are quite rational as adopters — with profit, risk, and opportunity cost all looming large in decisions to adopt.

While each counterargument questions the necessity of groups, the most powerful argument against organizing groups focuses on the improbability of doing so. The single strongest theme recurring through our review of extension activity, whether it be conventional or media based, is the complexity and difficulty of maintaining a field organization or a local group structure, even for the relatively small number of farmers who are directly reached by such systems. While there are exceptions, unless there is a long-standing cultural tradition of mutual aid (as in Taiwan or among the Tiv in Nigeria), field structures tend to atrophy. The promise of media-based projects is their ability to sidestep the requirement of field organization. If they lose that advantage because they depend on a parallel field channel, they may have little promise.

While we argue that media-based argricultural information projects cannot depend heavily on a parallel face-to-face communication channel to their target farmers, we do not suggest that they can function independently of field activities. On the contrary, what goes on in the field is of crucial importance.

Indeed, the major issue with regard to agricultural radio is having something useful to say to farmers in a given microclimate. If the agricultural economists are right, no media-based or conventional extension system will have a major effect on agricultural product much of the time. Most often they are ineffective, not because they are poor educational strategies, but because information, however presented, is not the appropriate solution. Other elements of what Arthur Mosher calls the Progressive Rural Structure are lacking, and throwing information at the problem is not going to help.

When, however, throwing information at a problem is a promising solution, because sharp changes in the resource environment of farmers make old practices less than optimal and new ones sufficiently rewarding, then broadcast approaches to extension are as promising as any others. Underlying this is the assumption that farmers are highly adaptive and ready to respond to new information if the economic incentives are right. Under this view, the primary problem of media-based diffusion systems is not in the technological system that diffuses the information but in the curriculum development/media production system that obtains and makes use of information from the field.

Of the media-based extension programs, open broadcast strategies for increasing agricultural productivity are more likely than any other promising method to be widely implemented (a key assumption that disqualifies most projects). They must, however, be linked closely with the field through an effective feedback system, be responsive to the actions of other agricultural agencies, and be realistic about the circumstances under which important increases in production can be achieved. Ideally they would be one element of a broader program of change, thus increasing the opportunity for information effects.

The cost of implementing such a system — even with a substantial staff charged with obtaining feedback from the field — should be far less than a conventional extension system per farmer reached. It has the potential for reaching many who do not have access to the conventional system under projected budgets. It is, of course, more expensive in terms of absolute budget than current agricultural broadcasting, but also should be more cost effective. We do not have evidence that such a system has actually worked. We do have important evidence (from BVE, Masagana 99, and elsewhere) that it is worth further trials, because it is both feasible and promising.

As for other uses of communication technology in the agricultural sector, our suggestions must be even more tentative. Investment in communication technology to enhance the distribution of market and weather information, to improve the management and support of field staffs where they are in place, and to develop channels of feedforward to increase the influence of farmers in the agricultural research process all seem to have potential, at least in the abstract. But investment decisions ought to await evidence that inadequate current flows of information are a substantial cause of existing failures in those areas.

In sum, conventional extension and group-dependent media-based projects are likely to be stymied by the improbability of developing field organizations that work, that reach large numbers of farmers, and that last. All programs to enhance information flows are likely to be constrained by the fact that information is only sometimes helpful since farmers are already responsive to perceived economic incentives. Where information is helpful (most likely when other changes in the farmers' environment are occurring simultaneously) open-broadcast strategies with a well-developed feedback system are as likely as any to affect agricultural practice change and productivity.

Part Three

Communication and Nutrition

Chapter Seven

The Roles of
Information in Nutrition

Malnutrition is widespread. According to the World Bank (1980), several hundred million people suffer from protein-energy malnutrition; hundreds of millions more suffer from the lack of certain micronutrients such as iron, iodine, and vitamin A. The human cost — in early death, in physical and possibly mental retardation, in debilitating illness, and in low energy levels that affect productivity — is awesome. The effects of malnutrition are particularly evident among very young children.

Many sources detail the nature and the consequences of this problem and examine alternative policy options for alleviating it (Berg 1981; Reutlinger and Selowsky 1976; World Bank 1980; USAID 1977). Many options focus on actions taken in the agricultural sector or in other programs to increase individual incomes. Some involve investments in community infrastructures (such as water treatment and electric power plants) or health systems. Others involve direct nutritional interventions such as food price subsidization, supplementary feeding programs, and the development of nutritionally improved foods. On most lists of potential policy options (sometimes near the bottom), one can also find nutrition education. The nutrition education option for combating malnutrition is the subject of Part Two of this book.

The central questions here are straightforward: Under what circumstances is there a role for nutrition education? In what content and behavior areas, with what educational methods, and for which populations is there evidence that education is an affordable, logistically feasible, and effective intervention? Can nutrition education stand on its own, or is it valuable exclusively as a component of a comprehensive nutrition intervention?

To answer these questions we need to establish three sequential conditions:

1. We need to show that there is a potential for nutrition education. We must show either (a) that currently available resources at the household level are not producing optimal nutritional benefit (that is, if people made better use of their current income they would be better fed), or (b) that current or coming changes in the environment (including noneducational nutrition interventions) could allow better nutritional status if people

knew how to adapt to those changes. If (a) can be established, it would be consistent with a nutrition education program standing alone. If only (b) can be established, then only nutrition education programs introduced in the context of naturally occurring or planned complementary changes can be justified. If neither (a) nor (b) can be established in a particular context, then nutrition education holds no potential.

2. We need to show that educational interventions can bring about desired changes in behavior and nutritional status. Saying that there exist materially feasible changes in behavior that are nutritionally beneficial is not the same as saying that a particular educational intervention can bring about those changes. We need to show that educational interventions have resulted in improved nutritional status.

3. Finally, we need to show that effective education can be realized on a scale that will benefit a large number of people. Of the three necessary conditions, this is the most difficult to establish. The inverse relation between effectiveness and scale, and ways to address that dilemma, will be major themes.

THE POTENTIAL FOR NUTRITION EDUCATION

The World Bank puts it bluntly: "Malnutrition is largely a reflection of poverty: people do not have enough income for food" (World Bank 1980, 59). Malnutrition is not a matter of a shortfall in aggregate agricultural production. Global food resources are more than sufficient to feed the world's population; indeed, in many nations where protein-energy malnutrition is common, there is enough food to feed everyone. Rather, malnutrition is largely a problem of equity; some people have incomes too small to purchase the food they require. This shortfall exists even though individuals are already spending a very high proportion of their income on food — 80 percent or more among the poorest half of the population in Indonesia, for example (World Bank 1980).

It is no surprise, then, that most sources turn outside the narrowly defined nutrition sector when suggesting solutions to malnutrition.

> Boosting food production (especially food that poor people eat and grow) and raising the incomes of the poor are the two central requirements in most countries (World Bank 1980, 62).

A commentator would be foolish to deny the primacy of the income-malnutrition link or its implications concerning the need for the equitable distribution of available food, if minimum adequate nourishment is to be enjoyed by all of a society's members. The next question becomes, Is there anything left over not determined by income? Is there nutritional inefficiency in the use of available resources? That is the key question in nutrition education.

Nutrition education seeks to enable consumers to use available resources optimally to reach valued ends. If current resources are already being used optimally, then nutrition education has no role. But knowing whether resources are being used optimally is no easy task. Optimality depends on one's weighting of the desired ends. One may value the survival and growth of children at weaning age and also the ability of adults to work without energy deficits. In some families, optimizing one end may be done only at the cost of the other.

Valued ends may include the desire to conform to community norms, personal convenience, avoidance of economic risk, acceptance of religious strictures, and so on. An argument that a particular practice is not optimal and thus is subject to nutrition education is as much a value judgment as a technical statement. It is a declaration about what ends should be sought as well as whether current resources are being used efficiently in achieving them. The issue is further complicated by considering whose ends — the beneficiaries' for themselves or the educators' for the beneficiaries — are to be chosen. Following this logic, we offer two categories of nonoptimality before we turn to the evidence for the optimality of particular nutrition-related behaviors.

1. *When current resources can be used more efficiently in obtaining a desired end without cost to other desired ends.* This is the easy case, in which nutrition education need only concern itself with providing information. If we can imagine a situation in which mothers choose to bottle-feed rather than breast-feed because they believe bottle feeding is nutritionally superior, there would be a logical possibility for changing behavior by changing what mothers know.

2. *When two desired ends are in conflict, and the nutrition educator believes that one ought to be valued over the other.* A mother may be aware that bottle feeding is less nutritionally valuable than breast feeding, yet choose the bottle for her infant because her "modern" social network expects her to. Nutrition education in this context becomes an attempt at persuasion, at convincing mothers to value one end over another. A closely related circumstance is when parents do not believe in a particular end that the nutrition educator values. Parents may not believe, for example, that weight-for-age growth is a definition of adequate nourishment. The nutrition educator who believes that it is needs to persuade parents to accept that criterion before teaching behaviors that will optimize it.

It is relatively easy to find situations in which current behavior is not optimal if outsiders are permitted to choose which ends are to be sought (category 2). It is harder to locate nonoptimal behavior when one accepts the existing values of the audience (category 1). The probability of finding exemplars of both these cases is greatly increased during times of substantial environmental change.

Evidence about educational potential comes from four sources: logical argument, expert testimony, empirical studies of dietary behavior, and studies of the effects of educational interventions. We first look at evidence about the potential for nutrition education at the aggregate household level and then turn to evidence about the potential for affecting nutrition within the household.

EDUCATION AT THE AGGREGATE HOUSEHOLD LEVEL

The conventional wisdom is that malnutrition at the aggregate household level is, for all practical purposes, defined by income. Knudsen and Scandizzo (1979) set the correlation between income and energy consumption per capita at about .95, based on their reading of data from six consumption surveys (from Bangladesh, India, Morocco, Sri Lanka, Pakistan, and Indonesia) using the household as the reporting unit. Their results say that, among the poorest people in the poorest countries, for each additional 10 percent of income there is a 7.5 percent to 8.5 percent increase in energy intake. These results leave little latitude for education in improving general household nutrition.

This position is not universally accepted, however. Behrman and Wolfe (1984) organize some confounding evidence, both from their own work in Nicaragua and from other studies. They find that in some countries and some poorly nourished groups, for each 10 percent increase in income there is less than a 4 percent increase in energy (and other nutrient) consumption. In Nicaragua they found an increase in calorie consumption of less than 1 percent with a 10 percent increase in income. They hypothesize that "even in a population with substantial malnutrition...this pattern may reflect...concern...with taste, convenience, status conferral and time intensity — as income increases." They are skeptical of the impact of increasing income on reducing malnutrition. By implication they suggest that improvements in nutritional status for many are possible with current resources and that educational interventions may hold promise.

These results are controversial and remain undeveloped with regard to specific implications for nutrition education. However, if they are confirmed, they may open substantial opportunities for educational interventions now viewed as closed by most observers. Nonetheless, even if we accept the assumption of a high correlation between income and energy consumption, we may find some ways in which education can resolve household-level malnutrition. First there is an argument that, energy aside, some nutrients *are* missing from typical diets, and not because of cost considerations. For example, vitamin A deficiency is common — 50 percent of the children in developing countries are said to suffer from it (World Bank 1980) — and some argue that it is remediable through the addition of small quantities of locally available foodstuffs or of the products of small home gardens.

Second, at a certain level of income some families consume more calories and are better nourished than others. While intraincome-level variation in energy consumption will not be enough to resolve the nutritional deficits of substantially impoverished families, households at the poverty line may show important variation in dietary adequacy. Thus, even a high correlation between income and energy consumption does not totally deny a role for nutrition education.

A related argument is that the income-energy correlation hides pockets of nonoptimal consumption. New urban migrants, refugees, and others have to make radical changes in dietary behavior; practices that previously took maximum advantage of available income may no longer be appropriate, given changes in income, in household structures, or in employment patterns. Similarly, the sudden availability of new foods or of changed prices for available foods may dictate changes in dietary behavior if maximum benefit is to be derived from available income.

A third argument is that calories purchased are not equivalent to calories utilized for nourishment. Food preparation and storage have important effects on nutritional benefits, both because nutritive value is directly affected and because the gastrointestinal illnesses associated with inadequate preparation and storage affect the utilization of available calories. Again, a potential role for education may remain.

While all of these arguments suggest possible roles for nutrition education, they do not necessarily indicate targets for nutrition education of the same magnitude as those that are addressed in the next section. Each argument refers to a special circumstance. Each justifies a particular directed educational effort if evidence shows that for a specific group the generally high correlation between income and nutritional status does not hold.

EDUCATION WITHIN THE HOUSEHOLD

If conventional wisdom is skeptical about the potential for education affecting aggregate household consumption, it is more enthusiastic concerning intrahousehold consumption. In Berg's view, "Sometimes...malnutrition occurs simply because food habits are inappropriate.... It is not uncommon, for example, to find children suffering from malnutrition in households in which incomes and food are adequate. Even among the poor, much childhood malnutrition could apparently be avoided" (1981, 26). Zeitlin and Formacion take a similar position: "A major proportion of this malnutrition [at weaning age] has been shown to be caused by ignorance, incorrect food and health beliefs, and resultant poor feeding and health practices, rather than lack of basic food resources" (1981, 4).

Evidence for the proposition that malnutrition is not entirely determined by income comes from a variety of sources. Perhaps the most common are descriptive studies of existing practices that are viewed implicitly or explicitly by their investigators as dysfunctional. The greatest number of these are anthropological studies of dietary behaviors of given cultural groups, often based on intensive observation of a relatively small sample of people. Many such studies are summarized and referenced in the *Maternal and Infant Nutrition Reviews* (*MINR*) prepared by the staff of the International Nutrition Communication Service and now available for Egypt, Lesotho, Liberia, Morocco, Nepal, Pakistan, Sri Lanka,

Tanzania, Thailand, Tunisia, and Zaire (Israel n.d.). These are very useful both for exploring specific practices within a given culture and for explaining the belief systems that underlie those practices. However, these studies do not provide estimates of how widespread a particular practice or belief is in a given country; they often suggest a greater universality of practices and explanations for practices than is in fact the case.

To obtain evidence about the extent of a given practice, one must turn to nutrition surveys that ask for (but often do not further validate) self-reports of current beliefs and practices. One recent survey done for CARE and reported by Vemury (1981) questioned randomly selected samples of rural mothers in six countries (Bangladesh, Colombia, Guatemala, Jordan, Peru, and Tunisia). Table 7.1 reports relevant practice data vis-à-vis several relevant themes from Vemury. We make use of specific data from this table in subsequent discussions.

These data (and the many smaller descriptive studies not summarized) do suggest that many apparently dysfunctional practices are widespread, although some are less common than has been suggested. If credible, the data support the argument for educational solutions, but in no sense are they conclusive. As has already been suggested, failure to act upon the optimal recommendations of outsiders may be due not to a lack of knowledge but to a conflict of values.

For each theme customarily addressed by nutrition educators, it is essential to ask how current behavior is best explained. Does the source of the behavior lie in lack of knowledge, preference for optimization of another value, or disinterest in maximizing a particular value? Is the behavior preferred by the outsider simply not feasible on economic grounds? We shall not examine these issues intensively for every nutritional theme; instead, we treat three problems and look at the existing knowledge concerning the explanations for each practice. We look at breast feeding among nonrural women (among rural women it is not so great a concern), the nutrition of weaning-age children, and the treatment of childhood diarrhea. Parallel analyses could have been undertaken for other behaviors often chosen by nutrition educators: the supplementation of diets of pregnant and lactating women, the production and use of vitamin A and protein sources, and improved sanitation, among others.

BREAST FEEDING AMONG NONRURAL WOMEN

Survey after survey reports that when asked why breast feeding was never instituted or not continued for very long, women reply that they had "insufficient milk." Since physiological inability is rarely found, most investigators seek explanations elsewhere. The hypotheses are many; we present them briefly and then look at the evidence for each.

- *Ignorance explanations*: Women do not understand the relative advantages of breast over bottle.
- *Medical system explanations*: Hospitals interfere with the development of the

TABLE 7.1 SELF-REPORTED NUTRITION BEHAVIOR —
VEMURY SIX-COUNTRY SURVEY

Issue	Peru	Colombia	Guatemala	Tunisia	Jordan	Bangla-desh
Feeding Preference — %						
Husband	57.3	52.6	45.5	73.0	27.0	64.0
Child under 6	4.3	8.2	.5	3.7	8.9	2.4
Not reported	4.2	27.7	48.3	12.1	40.1	5.3
Other	34.2	11.5	5.7	11.2	34.0	28.3
Harmful Foods						
Largest % naming any one food	*	*	*	11.0	4.0	12.0

(* — No food mentioned as harmful by more than 2% of the sample.)

Issue	Peru	Colombia	Guatemala	Tunisia	Jordan	Bangla-desh
Diet of Nursing Women						
% Who Report Eating						
More than normal	49.2	62.5	53.5	72.0	56.9	75.1
Normal	49.5	34.5	39.3	22.4	39.5	20.4
Less than normal	1.1	2.4	3.5	4.2	2.6	1.7
Initiation of Breastfeeding						
% Giving prelacteal feed	43.5	73.4	86.9	58.3	97.2	95.5
% Giving breast immediately	35.9	21.9	48.5	0.0	0.0	4.9
If not immediately, mean hours to initiation	25.7	34.0	16.4	46.6	62.2	62.1
% Who breastfeed	98.7	98.0	99.2	95.1	96.6	99.9
Mean months of breastfeeding	16.8	14.0	13.0	21.5	16.4	27.3
Treatment of Illness						
% Who:						
Withdraw breast if child is ill	47.6	41.3	40.0	41.8	34.7	60.5
Purge during diarrhea	11.6	8.3	16.3	2.1	3.4	9.1
Purge at unspecified times — possibly during diarrhea	0.0	64.7	36.1	81.1	21.7	27.3
Feeding Children						
% Who:						
Introduce foods before 6 months	72.9	81.5	63.7	43.9	66.3	59.4
(N)	(841)	(853)	(520)	(471)	(507)	(910)

sucking reflex by rigid and dysfunctional nursery practices; medical professionals work hand-in-hand with infant formula salespeople.
• *Marketing system explanations*: Women have learned to denigrate breast feeding as "unmodern," as a result of advertising campaigns and other social communication processes.

- *Economic explanations*: Women are working away from home in larger numbers; they are so malnourished themselves that they cannot support their infants.
- *Social psychological explanations*: Urban stress interferes with the letdown reflex; the lack of an extended family eliminates crucial social support and advice.
- *True preference explanations*: Women prefer bottle feeding for reasons of convenience (others can share bottle-feeding responsibilities), modesty (city people may be less accepting of public breast feeding than rural people), fear of loss of attractiveness, or desire to satisfy group norms.

Simple ignorance explanations are not consistent with the data now available. For example, surveys consistently find that women know that breast feeding is better than bottle feeding. While the true degree of advantage may not be universally understood, simple messages about comparative advantage, based on the assumption of ignorance in this area, are not likely to promise much change. Similarly, the elimination of pictures of healthy babies from the labels of evaporated milk cans (as pernicious as those are symbolically) is not likely to have much effect on the duration of breast feeding.

More complex misinformation is common. Many mothers have doubts about the quality of their milk and believe that some combination of breast and bottle is ideal. Premature supplementation, in turn, affects the mother's milk supply and may produce the common survey explanation for the end of breast feeding, "insufficient milk" (Sanghvi 1983; Valdivia 1983).

Existing data are somewhat ambiguous about the role of hospital practices (for example, the separation of newborns from mothers, the provision of prelacteal feeds, and delays in the initiation of breast feeding). Winikoff and Baer (1980) cite dozens of studies (but only a few in developing countries) demonstrating that changes in such hospital practices lead to changes in breast-feeding practice. The Jelliffes (1982) report that rooming-in, as part of the Brazilian national breast-feeding promotion campaign, produced higher rates of breast feeding, at least at the time mothers left the hospital.

It is difficult to know, however, whether these improvements reflect only the physiological effects of hospital practice. Psychological support by the hospital staff for breast feeding, which mothers could easily read from the changed practice, may also be important. In opposition to the purely physiological explanation, it appears that among the rural women in Vemury's surveys, who usually do not give birth in hospitals, quite long periods typically elapse before breast feeding is instituted (from 16 to 60 hours), and infants are customarily given some prelacteal feed (often sugar water) before being put to the breast. These practices are even more extreme than those common in hospitals and are cited as causes of failure to breast-feed. Nonetheless, breast feeding is successfully introduced and maintained among these rural women for many months. In fact, the Jelliffes also note that in Brazil the "common length of breast feeding in urban areas appears to be about sixteen days" (p. 22), which suggests that for most urban women the end of breast feeding comes well after leaving the hospital.

In sum, hospital practice may contribute to breast-feeding failure. It may make the first steps in establishing suckling and maintaining the mother's milk supply more difficult. When the mother is then turned out into an environment that does not make breast feeding easy, the shift to supplemental and then exclusive bottle feeding may occur more readily. However, improving hospital practices alone may not greatly increase the number of women who breast-feed for long periods of time.

Attacks on the infant formula marketing industry are widespread and a major concern of international conferences. Particular sales practices work against the best interests of mothers and their children, and much advertising of infant formula is morally offensive. What is unclear, however, is how strong a force such advertising is in the abandonment of breast feeding. Some recent evidence gives reason for skepticism.

There is a curious report from the Soviet Union, where such marketing is nonexistent but breast feeding nevertheless declines steadily (*Wall Street Journal* 1983). There are no reports of any substantial halt in the decline of breast feeding in some countries in which direct marketing activities have been restricted. There is the previously mentioned fact that women do not justify the use of formula on the grounds that it is as good for babies as breast milk, but rather because they had "insufficient milk." None of these reports supports the claim that formula advertising is a major cause of the decline in breast feeding. In any case, as a result of the passage of the WHO code, direct advertising of infant formula to mothers may be a thing of the past, at least in some countries (Post 1983). Indirect marketing through health professionals and point-of-sale displays remains common, although the Nestlé Company, the world's largest formula marketer, agreed in early 1984 to modify these practices.

What is no doubt true — even tautological — is that the availability of infant formula affects the probability of its use, and that restricting its availability will reduce its use. However, whether such restrictions will encourage breast feeding or reliance on even less-useful products, such as evaporated milk or cows' milk, is not so obvious.

Another hypothesis — that the decline in breast feeding is the result of women's increasing work roles — is not consistent with existing findings. Only a very small percentage of women across a large number of studies reported that work demands were responsible for early weaning (Van Esterik and Greiner 1981).

A major theme in current analyses attributes the cause of insufficient milk to a victory of urban stress and social dislocation over maternal self-confidence. This explanation is consistent with the sharp urban-rural differences in breast-feeding practice. According to the Jelliffes, this assumption underlies the Brazilian breast-feeding campaign and justifies information campaigns directed both toward mothers directly and toward health professionals in order to enable than to cope with isolated mothers' psychological and information needs.

An alternative view is also consistent with the data, if somewhat less promising for advocates of breast feeding. It falls in the category of true preference explanations. This view does not explain breast-feeding behavior in terms of the confidence levels of individual mothers or their specific knowledge about how to resolve problems that arise. Focusing on individual mothers and their success or failure is misleading; instead, within a social network, certain expectations for behavior are generated, based perhaps on what is typical in that group, perhaps on other forces. Those expectations may be communicated clearly to all who hold that network as reference group — particularly with regard to behavior that bears on the interaction of that network. If, for whatever reason, urban groups disapprove of lengthy breast feeding, individual mothers contravene those expectations only at some cost. This hypothesis suggests that the probability of a woman's breast feeding is best predicted by the breast feeding behavior of her five best friends.

Evidence in support of this view comes most sharply from the comparison of experiences over the last decades in more- and less-developed countries. Sanghvi (1983) makes the point clearly:

> At least some of the impetus and confidence among health professionals and policymakers in LDCs to take up the breast-feeding cause comes from this example [of more-developed countries]. With no noticeable mitigation in urban stress, change in family support and networks, or changes in trends toward women working outside the home, and increasing budgets for formula marketing and advertising, breast-feeding rates have increased and increased rapidly.

The implications of the group expectation explanation vis-à-vis the individual confidence and technical skill explanation for the viability of a nutrition education strategy are only somewhat clear. If norms rather than lack of skills lie at the heart of the issue, then emphasizing skills transmission is not likely to produce a major increase in breast feeding. Similarly, campaigns based on the assumption that non-breast-feeding mothers really want to breast-feed but lack the confidence may only have limited success. Their preferences may in fact be consistent with their behavior.

With regard to what should be done if group norms are predominant, two paths may be productive. From one perspective, a change in group norms is viewed as a long-term problem, one not likely to be affected by any thirteen-week, multichannel extravaganza, but by a much longer program of persuasive communication. Breast feeding must become the expected and institutionally supported behavior over the long term, with an understanding that the change in rates of breast feeding will be only gradual. A second possible path is a campaign designed to make breast feeding exempt from the influence of social networks. It may be that more latitude in individual choice is allowed in some types of behaviors than in others. For example, for urban, modern-aspiring women, any behavior required by the modern medical system might be exempt from social sanction. "The doctors say I have to" may justify otherwise unacceptable behavior. A campaign dedicated to making breast feeding a medically prescribed behavior may permit individual women to choose it. Such changes in individual behavior eventually may reshape social norms.

Obviously, much of this is only speculation and should be perceived as such. These explanations are certainly worth further discussion and empirical testing. However, the explanation for the decline in breast feeding that one accepts has profound implications for what, if any, strategy for nutrition education one adopts.

WEANING-AGE MALNUTRITION

There is is no question that failure to breast-feed is a major nutritional problem. The only mitigating factor in this nutritional problem is that it tends to skip the very poorest in most countries: rural children whose mothers almost always breast feed. The semi-urban and urban children whose mothers often bottle feed are sometimes from families who are a little better-off economically, and those children then have some chance to struggle back from malnutrition caused by bottle feeding. No such mitigating characteristic can be found for what is probably the largest problem of malnutrition: the failure of children aged 6 months to 4 or 5 years to get an adequate diet. Moderate to severe malnutrition among such children is found in most developing countries. The *MINR* reports suggest that the proportion of 6-to-60-month-old children who are malnourished (that is, whose weight is less than 75 percent of what it should be according to the Gomez age-weight classification) varies from 35 percent to 50 percent (Israel n.d.). The question is, How much of that is remediable, given the resources within households?

Dealing with this malnutrition involves three components: recognizing its presence, knowing how to combat it, and being able to take the required action. The first two are subject to nutrition education; the third places a limit on how much change is possible. There is, however, good reason to believe that a fair amount of change *can* take place before that limit is reached. A wide range of explanations for this type of malnutrition has been proposed. We list each and then describe them in detail, noting their implications for educational interventions. Explanations include:

- The pattern of intrafamily food distribution trades future growth of children for the current energy needs of income-earners.
- Childhood malnutrition serves, or has served, to control population growth. That effect was not counterbalanced, historically, by any mental skill advantage lent by adequate nutrition.
- A decline in extended breast feeding.
- A failure to recognize malnutrition.
- Ignorance about how to prepare nourishing foods from available sources.
- Continual pregnancies and the lack of time and energy to prepare special foods for weaned children.

- High infection rates and consequent reduced appetites and poor absorption of available nutrients.

Often it is suggested that the income-earning household members are given first preference at eating time. If there is meat or other high-protein/energy food, the income-earners are said to eat their fill, leaving only residual portions to others. Weaning-age children are given no preference at all. Certainly the Vemury survey data reported in Table 7.1 are consistent with that conclusion. In Peru, Colombia, Tunisia, and Bangladesh, more than half of the household respondents reported giving first preference to the husband, and almost none reported giving the most valued portion of the meal to the weaning-age child.

One obvious inference from such a result is that intrafamily food distribution follows a reasonable economic logic. Regardless of the long-term consequences for the health and productivity of the weaning-age child, the short-term consequences of depriving the income-earner of the energy required to earn that income may be extreme. As obvious as this may be, it turns out not to be consistent with the data.

If a conscious trade-off of current income-earner calories against future child growth is being made, several other statements should be possible. For families whose total energy availability exceeds household requirements, there should be adequate feeding of weaning-age children. Also, in energy-deficient families, underfeeding of children ought to occur at all ages up to the point when a child's ability to earn exceeds the marginal cost of providing the child with the additional calories necessary to permit the extra work activity. As noted by Zeitlin and Formacion, the findings of the Tamil Nadu nutrition study (Cantor and Associates 1973) directly contradict both of those statements.

Figure 7.1 summarizes the data of that study. It indicates that at one year of age, on the average, all children are ill-fed. Even children from families with surplus calories available receive less than 80 percent of their energy requirements. Indeed, only among those families with less than 70 percent of total necessary calories available to them is there any apparent equity of food distribution — the equity of borderline starvation. It also appears that the relative inequity disappears quite rapidly by the time a child is 3 years old, long before economic productivity can provide an explanation for the larger share being obtained.

The Tamil Nadu data make it clear that income alone does not explain the malnutrition of weaning-age children. While among the poorest of the poor, children and adults fare equally (and poorly), among the relatively better-off families, children are the victims of persisting dangerous and inequitable feeding practices.

This evidence presents a strange result. A clearly dysfunctional practice (if child survival and productivity are the desired ends) is maintained without producing any immediate countervailing advantage for the alternative end, the energy supply of the income-earner. It suggests that this practice represents a poor cultural adaptation in which people fail to obtain all that they can from meager resources. It promises, then, a wide-open field for nutrition education. Yet such a

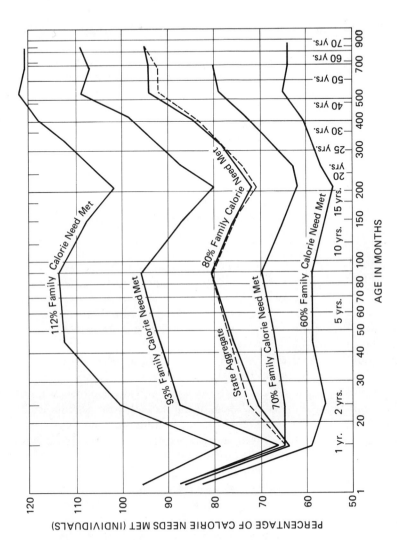

From Cantor and Associates, Inc. 1973, 101.

Figure 7.1. Percentage of Individual Calorie Needs Fulfilled, by Age, for Five Levels of Family Calorie Adequacy.

conclusion can be accepted only reluctantly. Too many "irrational" practices in other fields have turned out to be sensible adaptations to prevailing economic circumstances. In particular, it would be strange to find such an "irrational" practice common across so many cultures. And, in fact, a number of scholars have suggested that this pattern of feeding has had results that, while painful, have been functional over the long run for societal survival.

Cantor and Associates (1973) quotes Klein and his colleagues, "In oversimplified terms, death of pre-school children due to malnutrition is *de facto* the most widely used method of population control" (p. 34). Nutrition policy-planning documents (Knudsen 1981) customarily consider population growth effects in their calculation of the consequences of a nutrition intervention. Current practices have undeniable results, and the explanation of practices in terms of their results has a strong tradition in functional theories of anthropology and sociology. Susan Scrimshaw states the position most clearly when she says:

> When a certain level of infant mortality is "expected" or when a child is unwanted, there may be underinvestment in some children that is manifested in their care, their feeding, and the response to their illnesses (1978).

Indirect support for this position comes from Balderston's (1981) examination of the data from the INCAP protein supplement experiment in Guatemala and from the economic analyses of Selowsky (1981) and Knudsen (1981). They suggest that some positive benefits of adequate nourishment have been realized only recently. Historically those benefits may not have counterbalanced population control results. The supporting logic follows.

All of these sources argue that the economic benefit of improved mental skills possibly associated with the better feeding of preschool children is dependent on obtaining complementary formal education. In an earlier period when there was no formal schooling (nor opportunity to make use of the skills that formal education provided), the economic benefit to better-nourished children may not have been very large. The recent work of Lockheed and her associates (1980) extends this hypothesis. They found large increases in agricultural productivity associated with additional education but only in rapidly changing agricultural environments. In static environments, better-educated and less-educated farmers fared equally. By analogy, if in an earlier period static agriculture was the norm, the economic return on enhanced intellectual capacities due to better nourishment may have been minimal. If so, the economic benefits of improved nutrition may not have counterbalanced the population control results.*

---

* Evidence for the association between mild and moderate malnutrition and intellectual capacity on which this hypothesis depends is by no means unequivocal. Certainly, height predicts achievement (Balderston et al. 1981), and one form of malnutrition is defined by height-for-age (Griffiths 1981). However, whether those height/malnutrition and height/achievement correlations are sufficient grounds for a causal inference about the effects of malnutrition on achievement or intellectual capacity is an open question (Habicht 1983).

Nonetheless, even if these explanations (population control and lack of reward for intellectual capacity) did define the historical origins of current practice, they may no longer explain the continuation of this practice in some places. Materialist origins of a practice may disappear, yet the residual practice is maintained. As the environment changes (if it does) and rewards intellectual skills and provides alternative paths to population control, the residual behavior legitimately may be seen as maladapted. Perhaps the best evidence that current behavior is *not* well adapted comes from the studies that show that the dangerous feeding practices outlined in Table 7.1 are, in fact, subject to modification through educational intervention. Several studies show declines in malnutrition as the result of educational interventions alone — a result inconsistent with the hypothesis that current practice is well adapted. (We examine those studies in Chapter 8.) However, if these material explanations for current behavior are inadequate, it is necessary to turn to alternative explanations. Some, but not all, of these alternative explanations will suggest potential roles for nutrition education.

Given the current decline in breast feeding, might it be that a significant portion of weaning-time malnutrition is the result of the failure to replace breast milk with equivalent foods? This is not consistent with the data. Most malnutrition occurs after six months and at that time is more, rather than less, likely to be found among children who still depend on breast milk. One of the major problems associated with post-six-month malnutrition is the failure to supplement breast milk with solid foods and not the failure to maintain breast feeding.

Other explanations exist for the underfeeding of children. To some degree, parents cannot recognize malnutrition, particularly when it involves weight-for-age. In Zaire, 10 percent of a sample of mothers reported their children malnourished, whereas 32 to 47 percent actually were malnourished (Israel: Zaire n.d.). Zeitlin and Formacion describe a similar finding in the Philippines, where nearly 40 percent of the mothers of children suffering second- and third-degree malnutrition thought "their babies were growing and developing well" (1981, 69). This is not a surprising finding, given Zeitlin and Formacion's conclusion, "the average malnourished child in the 6- to 24-month age range cannot be identified without a weighing scale" (p. 68). If malnourishment is as widespread as the statistics suggest, the commonness of low weight-for-age is likely to lead parents to the conclusion that their children are at the norm.

It is possible that some parents fail to recognize malnutrition because they are unwilling to admit publicly that their child is malnourished, especially if no resources are available to remedy the problem. However, for the moment it is reasonable to assume that most simply do not recognize malnutrition when they see it. Children between 60 and 75 percent weight-for-age make up the bulk of the seriously malnourished, and they escape notice, despite the significant probability of long-term effects on productivity (Selowsky 1981; Knudsen 1981) and on health and susceptibility to disease (Rosenberg 1976, as quoted in Balderston et al. 1981; Berg 1981).

Whatever the origin of poor feeding of weaning-age children, a major block to the improvement of their nutritional status may be ignorance of how to prepare appropriate foods. Nutritionally adequate adult foods may be seen as too harsh for small children and thus withheld, but customarily used paps may lack nutritional quality, particularly energy density. Parents may be unaware of methods for making paps nutritionally adequate or adult foods more digestible.

However, failure to prepare special foods may not be the result of inadequate knowledge alone, a point incorporated in an explanation for malnutrition offered by Gretel Pelto (1981). She notes that the 6- to 12-month postnatal period coincident with much malnourishment is often a time of renewed pregnancy, with its sometimes debilitating side effects for a mother. Obviously this is a less than ideal moment for an infant to be making demands on its mother's time with requirements for specially prepared food in addition to breast feeding.

Another major explanation for much of the malnutrition among 6- to 24-month-old children may not turn on underfeeding at all (Chen and Scrimshaw 1983). Six months is the age of the onset of greater mobility and of partial weaning. It is a time of extraordinary increases in exposure to infection. The large number of diarrheal episodes and other infections are accompanied by loss of appetite and other stresses that may contribute to growth retardation. Normal feeding may not be enough to replace the protein and energy lost through the diarrhea, through the accompanying loss of absorptive capacity and anorexia, and through stress-related protein loss. This means that the actual protein and energy requirements for small children will be much greater than standard FAO (1974) requirements. In evaluating a recent study in Indonesia, Zeitlin (1984) followed the recommendation of N. Scrimshaw and estimated that 6- to 24-month-old children require 50 percent additional protein, and infants up to 6 months require 30 percent additional protein above the FAO estimates in order to counteract the effects of infection. The transfer of energy and protein resources from the rest of the family to the weaning-age child may need to be considerably greater than standard nutrient tables suggest.

This analysis suggests that the apparent undersupply of calories presented in the Tamil Nadu figure tells only part of the story, and that the actual percentage of necessary calories received by children in this age group is less than the 60 percent to 70 percent reported there. It supports the conclusion of the Guatemala INCAP experiments that consumption of a full share of calories by children reduced growth retardation only by one third. The rest of the children's growth retardation was said to reflect morbidity and factors other than energy consumption (Martorell, Habicht, and Klein 1982; Martorell 1984).

We are left with a series of explanations for weaning-age malnutrition. Part of it is explained by lack of income and poor intrafamily food distribution. Part of it may be the reflection (or the residual) of societal functions like population control and the lack of rewards for having rapidly growing children. If in a particular environment these adaptations are no longer necessary, nutrition education may be appropriate in correcting residual practice. Part of this kind of malnutrition reflects anorexia associated with morbidity, a subject to be looked at in terms of the potential for educational intervention in the next section.

A final explanation combines the family's failure to recognize mild and moderate malnutrition, its lack of knowledge about suitable weaning foods, and its lack of time and energy to give special attention to the needs of the weaning child. All three may be subject to nutrition education, although if time committed to the 6- to 24-month-old is to be increased, education may face a difficult path.

In sum, what does all of this say about the potential for nutrition education with regard to infant-feeding practice? Nutrition education is unlikely to be a complete solution in many contexts where income and time are particularly short. In other contexts, however, better practice will be consistent with available resources and subject to educational interventions.

NUTRITIONAL TREATMENT OF DIARRHEA

The third area we have chosen to examine is nutritional treatment during episodes of diarrhea. Diarrheal episodes are frequent among children in developing countries and a major cause of malnutrition and death. Whether or not much can be done about the incidence of diarrhea is not at issue here, although some may argue that educational interventions are potentially worthwhile. Of immediate concern is the nutritional consequences of diarrheal episodes and the potential for reducing those consequences through educational intervention. Three obvious points of intervention are worth consideration; they include treatment of dehydration through administration of oral rehydration salts (ORS) solution, avoidance of deleterious practices (like purging or the withdrawal of breast milk), and positive efforts to encourage feeding in the presence of poor appetite.

The potential for education in the first of these, ORS, is by far the strongest. ORS is efficacious if administered appropriately; it is within the resources of almost all (particularly the home-mixed sugar and salt solution); its preparation and administration can be mastered. Mothers often can recognize the signs of dehydration and, seeking remedies for the diarrhea they know to be a threatening condition, are willing to purchase even expensive treatments from pharmacies and traditional healers (Smith et al. 1980).

Yet there are problems too. Home-mixed ORS fluid can be toxic if it is prepared with incorrect proportions of sugar and salt or too little liquid; the latter is also a risk with packaged mixes. It has to be administered slowly, in substantial quantities, over a long period. It may appear to exacerbate the symptoms of diarrhea. While effective in the long run and at an aggregate community level, the odds that a particular treatment of ORS will save a life are quite small, since the proportion of episodes of diarrhea that lead to death is quite small. All of these problems, while they do not negate the potential for an educational intervention, may make the task of achieving effective practice change much more difficult.

The second major point of entry is in education concerning the avoidance of deleterious practices. Most attention is given to purging as a method for treating diarrhea, with its exacerbation of dehydration, and to the withdrawal of food, including breast milk, during episodes, particularly if the diarrhea is accompanied by vomiting. The natural logic of both of these actions is clear — purges because they "clean the system out," and withdrawal of food and liquid because it gives the digestive system a rest and reduces the diarrhea. Yet both, according to current medical opinion, are harmful and need to be eliminated.

However, before major educational efforts are mounted, it may be worth ascertaining whether these negative practices are in fact widespread. There is substantial ambiguity about this point. In his six-country CARE survey, Vemury found that purging was common in general but rare during episodes of diarrhea. Similarly, few mothers in those surveys reported withdrawal of the breast during episodes of diarrhea. In contrast, in Honduras, Foote and his colleagues (1983) found that close to 70 percent of a rural sample would name a specific purgative when asked how they treated a child's most recent instance of diarrhea, and 66 percent reported they withheld the breast. It may be that this contradiction is merely the result of cultural differences between Honduras and the countries Vemury surveyed. However, differences in the way questions were asked is a more likely explanation. If the Vemury results can be believed and generalized, a great deal of education may not be necessary on these topics. In contrast, if Foote's results are accepted in a particular context, they may justify a major educational effort.

The third point of educational entry is the taking of positive steps to ensure that children suffering from diarrhea get as much nourishment as possible. Failure to feed may be the result of deliberate withholding of the breast or other foods. More commonly, underfeeding may be the result of disinterest in eating on the part of the sick child. Usual feeding practices may need to be modified, including smaller feedings at more frequent intervals and the offering of specially prepared foods. Oral rehydration fluids may have a positive effect on the child's appetite as well. The degree of interaction between diarrhea (and vomiting, when it occurs), reduced appetite, parental unwillingness to feed a child (sometimes supported by medical advice), efficacy of alternative feeding practices and parental knowledge of them, time required of caretakers to feed a sick child effectively, and complementary effects of rehydration is likely to be large. Obviously educational interventions have potential only insofar as reduced appetite is not an absolute constraint, and families can reallocate time to the feeding of these children. Despite the magnitude of this problem and the efforts to address it as part of a broader program, little detailed evidence has been reported.

The potential for beneficial change in child-feeding practices during diarrheal episodes may be real and subject to education. However, the paucity of codified project experience limits further discussion of this. Arguments in favor of educational potential rely on their surface logic. Stronger arguments await evidence of what determines feeding practice during illness.

This exploration of the potential for nutrition education is not as definitive as we might have wanted. This is partly the result of thin research but it also reflects the difficulty of crosscultural generalization. What may be open to education in one culture may be closed to it in others. However, those considerations do not eliminate all potential for nutrition education. In the end, the best evidence for such a potential turns out to be the successful realization of an educational program. If a program has been able to change nutritional status through nutrition education, then there must have been the potential to do so. It is to the evidence from such realizations that we turn now.

Chapter Eight

On the Possibility of Doing Nutrition Education

Nutrition education is a common activity. Ninety-one percent of the 201 nutrition programs in 66 countries surveyed by the Harvard Institute for International Development (Austin et al. 1978) reported undertaking some type of nutrition education. Even so, most nutrition education is likely to have been missed by that extensive survey, since it tended to concentrate on discrete nutrition projects; it would probably have skipped the largest volume of nutrition education, which is undertaken as a routine activity of health workers.

The description and evaluation of nutrition education activity is, however, rarer than its practice. There may also be an inverse relation between the commonness of a type of nutrition education and the number of descriptions or evaluations of it. Not surprisingly, evaluations often focus on novel small-scale efforts and ignore ongoing routine activity. This may be a reflection of a belief that such ongoing activity has no important effects, or it may be a reflection of the nature of evaluation funding arrangements that focus on discrete projects. Thus we have a fair number of evaluations and descriptions of projects that use media or that incorporate face-to-face education in a special way, but essentially none for the rountine education undertaken by health services. This lack is a substantial concern. A reasonable number of evaluations now provide credible evidence for the positive effects of nutrition education on nutritional status. What is lacking is evidence about the feasibility of reproducing those results routinely and on a large scale.

Full descriptions of conventional nutrition education projects would also have helped us organize the review that follows. Ideally, we would have liked to describe the operation of a current typical system and then point out its flaws. Such flaws would have highlighted the presentation of alternative strategies, which would have been described in terms of the problems in the conventional system they were trying to solve. Indeed, such an approach is so attractive that we have decided to create a conventional system by supposition and then point out its likely problems. We can only hope that our "straw" system does not overly distort actual practice, or at the very least that its helpfulness as a convenient stereotype justifies its use.

A HYPOTHETICAL CONVENTIONAL SYSTEM
AND ITS FLAWS

In this system, nutrition education takes place essentially within the walls of a health clinic. Mothers bring their children in for curative services but on the walls are posters encouraging breast feeding and immunization (and a blank space where the poster supplied by the infant formula company used to be). The professional health staff are expected to provide general health and nutrition education in response to problems that individual mothers present. During the few minutes that the professional examines a malnourished child, the mother is counseled to give more food. The professional supplies other advice as he or she has time and believes it to be appropriate for particular mothers. The advice is drawn from the few days of classes concerning nutrition education received during the professional's medical training. Little follow-up on the implementation of the education is undertaken. Little change in nutritional status is achieved.

The result is ineffective nutrition education, but what specific problems need remedying? The list includes audience reach and time of exposure to education, quality and systematicness of education, reinforcement of messages, complementary environmental change, incentives for professionals, and cost.

Audience Reach. By relying on people to visit clinics, a nutrition education system may reach only a small proportion of the population. A large number of people, including many of the most malnourished, may not be served by those clinics, and many of those that are served may attend only irregularly. In addition, the few minutes of professional time in the clinic are unlikely to be enough to provide new skills, even if they had any influence on knowledge.

Quality and Systematicness of Education. Haphazard instruction, based on long-ago training, by professionals qualified as care providers, not as educators, is unlikely to prove effective. Content may not build on what mothers already know and do, or it may advocate practices that their socioeconomic circumstances do not allow them to undertake. Teaching may ignore the need to practice newly learned skills or may offer no concrete recommendations.

Reinforcement of Messages. Information about appropriate nutrition-related practice comes from many sources other than the clinic professional: from one's family and neighbors, from radio advertisements, and from retail displays and shopkeepers. Education derived from a clinic professional during a single visit may have little effect if contradictory messages are pouring in from other sources in the environment.

Complementary Environmental Change. Sometimes it is possible to affect nutritional status by education alone; often it is not. In recognition of this, many programs combine education with "real" changes such as food supplementation.

Similarly, even if an educator's recommendations would be effective if adopted, it may be necessary to combine education with other, more-demanded services if an audience is going to be persuaded to accept the education. (That is the reason why education is so often delivered in the context of curative health services, which bring in the audiences.)

Incentives. In the first three weeks in the field, after a sufficiently enthusiastic set of lectures on the utility of nutrition education, the health worker may initiate improved nutrition education. Yet the health clinic provides few incentives to maintain that enthusiasm; demands for time in curative medicine are large, and nutrition education is just a supplementary duty. No one comes around and checks on the number of hours of nutrition education delivered, or provides advice on how best to do it. No salary increments accrue for success in this area. Unsurprisingly, most health workers find it difficult to maintain their enthusiasm in such circumstances.

Costs. Using highly trained health professionals for some nutrition education activities can be a very expensive use of time. Weighing and measuring children in order to teach mothers to recognize malnutrition, providing instruction in food preparation, and other mainstays of nutrition education curricula are not necessarily better done by professionals than by less highly trained personnel. The haphazardness of nutrition education in the clinic setting may itself be a reflection of the cost of reallocating expensive professional time to a task for which such training is not suitable. Any attempts to extend the reach of nutrition education or increase the time of exposure face the major obstacle of financing.

SOLVING PROBLEMS OF THE CONVENTIONAL MODEL: PAST EXPERIENCE

We next turn to specific projects that have attempted to redress one or more of these failures. Descriptions of individual projects are presented as illustrations of the way they address a given problem. Many projects, of course, serve as potential solutions to more than one failure; these are described at the place where they provide most insight. To avoid redundancy, some projects that serve functions parallel to others are not described fully.

Audience Reach and Time of Exposure
If much of the malnourished population lies outside the reach of the formal health care system, clinic-based nutrition education cannot touch it. Attempts to extend the reach of the nutrition education effort follow several strategies, sometimes in combination. They include sending outreach workers to the homes of potential clients, using mass media, and providing new incentives for people to come to clinics (often by distributing subsidized food).

Outreach Programs. If the clients will not come to the clinic, then the clinic must reach out to the clients. The Promotora Program in Candelaria, Colombia, is an example of the attempt to reach out from the clinic to the malnourished population. Ten young women with a minimum of five years of education were given six months of specialized training. They were sent out to make regular visits in a small area to all families with children under two years of age. They provided "education on nutrition, hygiene, and utilization of health services; gathered data, including child height and weight; and referred sick children to a Health Service Unit" (Drake et al. 1980, 1). The young women were volunteers (presumably unpaid). The program continued for six years, from 1968 to 1974, as did the first phase of the evaluation. Similar programs have been described for Thailand (Viravaidhya et al. 1981), and Hanover, Jamaica (Gwatkin, et al. 1980).

The Hanover program was far larger than the Colombian one, serving a total population of 60,000 with 150 paid health aides. In the Colombian program, it appears that every family, regardless of the presence of malnourished children (ninety-two families for each aide), was visited every two months. In contrast, in Hanover, a preliminary screening located malnourished children, and then families with malnourished children were visited at least weekly. Calculations based on data presented in Gwatkin and associates (1980) suggest that each Hanover aide was responsible for eighteen malnourished children. The combination of screening and intensive visits to malnourished children's families is, on the surface, a productive way of concentrating resources on those most in need. It risks, of course, leaving out those children and families that do not qualify for intensive visits on the basis of malnourishment but would be in need of the extended health surveillance on other grounds.

The reports of three of these projects (Hanover, Candelaria, and Thailand) provide some evidence of positive effect of outreach programs on nutritional status and other outcome variables, although the conclusions are equivocal. The strongest result occurs in the Hanover project, where second- and third-degree malnutrition declined by 40 percent to 50 percent after a year of activity.

The Candelaria project evaluation provides positive short-term results and ambiguous longer-term evidence. The presence of the project coincided with a 25 percent drop in all malnutrition in the community between 1968 and 1974, despite relatively high turnover among participating families. Longer enrollment in the program was associated with even larger drops in malnutrition rates. The gains in nutritional status occurred despite erosion of family income during the period, and may have been related primarily to a reduced incidence of diarrhea. All of this was certainly positive evidence. However, a two-year follow-up study of effects sounded a note of caution. The project itself had been terminated in 1974, and researchers returned in 1976 to investigate the residual effects of the program. They found that children born after the end of the program into families that had participated were no better off than children in families that had not participated. Older children seemed to show some residual effect of their participation in the program.

The Thailand project showed a substantial drop (from 22 percent to 9 percent over six months) in second- and third-degree malnutrition in one town in which nutrition surveillance and nutrition education activities were carried out by village workers, and much smaller drops in control towns and in towns where only nutrition surveillance had taken place. The study is described only briefly, and possible threats to the inference of success (for example, changes in measurement quality, other current activities) are not fully considered. However, the results are consistent with those of the Hanover and Candelaria studies.

The costs of realizing these projects are not shown in the relevant sources. However, they obviously vary with the use of volunteers or paid staff, the amount of training and supervision provided by health professionals, the intensity of surveillance and education actually undertaken, the focus on vulnerable segments of the audience or on all its members, and the physical concentration of the families to be reached. As a solution to the problem of audience reach, these projects must be regarded as a potential strategy, but subject to important real-world limitations.

At the rate of eighteen malnourished children per paid health worker (the standard for the Jamaica project), the absolute budgetary requirement can be huge, particularly in those poor countries where the malnourishment problem is largest and national budgets smallest. Even in projects like the Candelaria activity, which depended on infrequent home visits of volunteer workers, the budgetary requirements are substantial. A volunteer-based program assumes an in-place health service infrastructure that provides both training of volunteers and most of the necessary health care. In many countries, the health services are located at great distances from much of the population; in Zaire, for example, only 25 percent of the population has access to the formal health care system (Israel: Zaire, n.d.). There are too few health clinics from which outreach workers can reach out. Volunteers workers also tend to turn over with some rapidity, with major cost implications for training and supervision activities.

Budgetary limits on the expansion of these outreach programs will be substantial. Nonetheless some countries may be willing to pay their cost if sufficient reduction in malnourishment can be achieved. However, a second type of limitation may be even more difficult to eliminate. Both the Hanover project and the Candelaria project were attempts by outside agencies to focus highly paid energies on the development of pilot activity. Hanover relied on help from the University of the West Indies and from Cornell University Medical School. Candelaria was the field site for a number of projects from the Universidad del Valle in Cali, including a rural health teaching center. When that first novelty dissipates and it becomes time for the creation of a national, long-term, routine program based on these models, they can no longer depend on that special energy. They must depend instead on internal incentives to operate effectively. We do not have any evidence that such "real" programs are effective. However, a comment from the authors of the Thai study is revealing in this context.

> During recent years the Royal Thai Government's Ministry of Public Health has initiated many new programs to deal with infant and pre-school nutrition. These programs include: supplemental feeding programs;...establishing child nutrition centers; nutrition education for mothers;...promotion of breast feeding; training in nutrition for village health volunteers and village health communicators; and limited nutrition surveillance. However a comparison of 1977 malnutrition data with 1980 age/weight data indicates no progress has been made (Viravaidhya et al. 1981, 1).

These activities, or a subset of them (surveillance and weighing), were the same as those that were undertaken in the experimental study, the positive results of which have already been presented. The essential difference between what had been done in the past without effect and what was being done in the evaluated project seems to have been the level of supervision and the presence of the investigators from the central Ministry of Health. The contrast may suggest the difficulty of transferring an activity that can be done successfully on a small scale to a large-scale national program. One other project, the World Bank Indonesia Nutrition Education program, has much in common with these programs and shows similar success. However, it will contribute more at a later point in the narrative, and thus its presentation is delayed.

If financial and logistical obstacles constrain the potential of outreach strategies, there are other approaches worth considering. The largest number of them make use of mass media.

Mass Media Alone. The "magic multipliers," as advocates are fond of calling the mass media, have often seemed to be the ideal way of solving the immense problems of reaching large audiences. In the face-to-face outreach system, each additional client costs the central government about as much to serve as does each previous client. In a mass-media-only system, the marginal cost to the government can be close to zero for each client after the first. Additional costs are funded directly by the client in the purchase price and energy expenditure of the privately owned radio.

Media-based nutrition education projects are legion. In the survey of nutrition projects previously cited (Austin et al. 1978), more than 25 percent of all projects reported using radio or television as channels for education. Thus media-based projects are common and, in some cases, evaluations of them are also available. However, none of those evaluations makes a convincing case for the effectiveness of media in changing nutritional status. Sometimes that is because the evidence shows no effects. More often, it is because the evaluations lack adequate evidence on which to base a confident judgment. Results from the ORS promotion projects in Egypt, Honduras, The Gambia, and Swaziland, discussed subsequently, will provide good evidence about practice change, but they do not provide evidence about nutritional status change. What existing evaluations do provide is data relevant to determining the effectiveness of media-based education systems in solving some of the hypothetical failures of conventional systems, including evidence about reach.

From the very first efforts at using mass media for nutrition education, it was clear that audiences could be reached, if reach is taken to mean gaining attention. An early evaluated effort at media-based nutrition education occurred in the Republic of Korea in 1970 under CARE sponsorship. A year-long campaign, it included twice-daily radio spots and a calendar and a comic book, which were produced and distributed. The main focus of the campaign was on the achievement of a balanced diet and, subsequently, on the use of solid weaning foods for children more than 100 days old. The evaluation was limited to a postcampaign survey of a sample of unspecified origin and contained no useful information about effectiveness. It did suggest that the campaign gained the attention of much of the population, with close to 90 percent of both urban and rural persons surveyed demonstrating some awareness of the existence of campaign materials. Memory of specific campaign messages was rather less (20 percent to 50 percent) and limited primarily to younger, well-educated middle-class respondents (Higgins and Montague 1972).

Similar evidence of effectiveness of reach comes from another CARE–sponsored campaign — this time over a ten-week period — in India. Multiple channels were used in this 1972 project in Uttar Pradesh and Andhra Pradesh, and its evaluation described large changes in the areas of knowledge related to weaning-food practice (an increase from 59 percent knowledgeable before the campaign to 93 percent after) and in general nutrition knowledge (72 percent to 96 percent) (CARE 1973; Rasmuson 1977). Both sampling procedures and methods of questioning may have created some bias in these results, but the effectiveness of the intensive media campaign in reaching an audience is probably credible.

Additional evidence of the reach of nutrition education broadcasting comes from reports about a different use of radio, in programs in Sri Lanka, Costa Rica, and Haiti. In all three countries, government agencies developed ten- to twenty-minute health information programs that relied on entertainment broadcasting formats. In each case, the radio dramas ("Pahan Siluwa" and "Kan Kanda Theivam") of Sri Lanka, and the programs of dialogue with a knowledgeable person of Costa Rica ("Pláticas con Don Rafael") and Haiti ("Radio Docteur") were skillfully produced programs that apparently reached wide audiences. Exact reach was never estimated for any of them in a formal survey, but on the basis of small surveys and of the sheer volume of letters and postcards received, the assumption of large audiences is credible. However, no useful information about what was learned from these programs (let alone changes in practice or nutritional status produced by them) is available (Burke et al. 1980; Clearinghouse on Development Communication 1980).

Until quite recently, the most sophisticated efforts using mass media were three projects conducted by Richard K. Manoff International, Inc. Manoff is a United States advertising firm that argued that it could apply Madison Avenue advertising techniques in order to change nutrition-related behavior in developing countries. Under contract with the U.S. Agency for International Development, Manoff developed projects in Ecuador (Manoff International 1976) and in Nicaragua and the Philippines (Cooke and Romweber 1977; Zeitlin and Formacion 1981). These projects prepared and arranged the broadcast of commercial spots recommending a particular nutrition behavior. Each series was broadcast repeatedly, up to 10 times per day over a period as long as a year. The themes covered depended on local conditions: in Ecuador, they included promotion of the use of iodized salt and of boiled water; in the Philippines, the early use of weaning foods and their supplementation with oil, fish, and vegetables; in Nicaragua, the use of an oral rehydration formula called *superlimonada* to combat dehydration.

The intensive broadcasts of well-produced spots clearly attracted a large audience. In the Philippines, up to 75 percent of the audience reported awareness of radio messages, and up to 65 percent of the audience reported a similar awareness in Nicaragua. Some evidence of knowledge and attitude change was found in all three countries. Behavior changes related to nutritional status were not so conclusively demonstrated.

In Ecuador, iodized salt replaced refined salt without iodine to a substantial degree, but no change in other recommended behaviors was apparent. In the Philippines, where the objective was to increase energy consumption at weaning time, self-reported changes in behavior did occur. For example, about one fourth of the sample reported adding oil to *lugaw*, a local weaning food, after the campaign, while none had reported doing so beforehand. (We will leave aside issues of the validity of self-reports of behavior that respondents knew was "right" according to radio broadcasts.) Even taken at face value, the behavior change actually reported (in terms of number of calories added to weaning food) was very small in relation to actual deficit, even among those who were classified as adopters of the new behavior. Again, in Nicaragua, while there was a self-reported increase in the use of the recommended rehydration formula, there is no evidence that it was used in sufficient quantities to affect dehydration and its consequences.

In their very full review of the Manoff Philippines project, Zeitlin and Formacion take the position that the failure to affect nutritional status was not a failure of the radio strategy per se. They suggest that if messages had been adjusted to reflect circumstances in the rural areas more closely (by recommending that oil be added to foods other than lugaw that were more commonly given to children), the program might have been effective. The need for a closer and continuing tie between producer and client in order to make mid-project adjustments feasible is an issue we shall take up in a subsequent section. It may be seen as the major change between these Manoff projects and the Mass Media Health Practices Project and the Manoff-implemented Indonesia project.

Large audiences may well be reached by media-alone projects. (Further supporting data come from projects in Honduras and The Gambia [Foote et al. 1986], in Swaziland [Hornik and Sankar 1986], and the Dr. Hakim project in Tunisia [Smith 1979].) However, broadcasting does not always guarantee attention, particularly when there are other competing messages. While reports of programs that failed to reach an audience tend not to be published, some such reports are available.

Among its other efforts, the Satellite Instructional Television Experiment in India tried to present nutrition education on some of its evening broadcasts. The only available evaluation of it suggested that the audience was so small as to make any assessmemt of effectiveness pointless. Only 36 out of 489 women in the two sample villages viewed the telecasts whose effects the evaluators wished to estimate. A variety of explanations for the failure to view were offered (language, motivation, alternative tasks to complete, poor-quality programming), but the point that an available audience does not guarantee an attending audience is clearly made (Ramadasmurthy et al. 1978). Relatively small audiences have also been described for a Brazilian nutrition education program using radio and for a two-week radio campaign in Lesotho (Leslie 1977). In another context, the "Feeling Good" television series, the major recent effort in the United States to provide health and nutrition education via the mass media, failed altogether to gain an audience, even by the minimal standards of the Public Broadcasting System, and was quickly cancelled.

There is one frequently raised objection to the assumption that radio broadcasts can effectively reach much of the rural population. Radio ownership is not universal, nor are the funds to keep radios working. In addition, ownership is least likely among the poorest segment of the population, who are also most likely to be subject to malnutrition. Three responses to this objection may be offered. First, radio ownership, particularly in Latin America and much of Asia, is still more widespread than is access to health systems. Radio ownership in rural areas was typically around 50 percent of all households, with some variation (Shore 1980). In countries with shortwave rather than medium-wave (AM) broadcasts to rural areas, coverage may be somewhat less. (In Nepal, for example, about 10 percent of all families had radios [Mayo et al. 1975].) Second, there is likely to be substantial access to radio among nonowners. They may have the opportunity to listen to radios in public places or in owners' houses. (Thus in the Manoff Philippines study only 48 percent of respondents owned radios but 75 percent reported being aware of radio messages.) Finally, even those who may not have an opportunity to hear messages directly are likely to hear them secondhand from listeners.

Perhaps the largest single obstacle to access to radio broadcasts is not the inability to buy a receiver or even batteries to keep it running, but rather problems of language. In India, in much of Africa, and in the indigenously populated regions of Central and South America, where many languages are spoken, even moderate efforts at multilingual programming may miss large numbers of people. The problem is exacerbated when women are the primary audience for broadcasts, since they are often less likely than men to understand outside languages. Another factor that complicates easy reach of target audiences through radio is the tendency, in some cultures, for one member of the family to control the use of the household radio. For example, O'Sullivan (1980) reports that in Guatemala men often take radios with them to the fields during the workday. Another problem is the competition for the listener's attention from multiple radio stations. This is particularly severe in Latin America, where the commercial character of the radio system has meant a proliferation of radio stations (Lee 1980), and in border areas of countries whose neighbors have strong transmitters, as is the case with the Indian state of Tamil Nadu and nearby Sri Lanka broadcasts (Green 1983), and with southern Nepal and All-India Radio (Mayo et al. 1975) Attention is also threatened when nationally funded radio programs are restricted to donated time from private stations or are assigned time on government-owned stations. It may turn out to be difficult to obtain much listener attention if the assigned times and frequencies are not convenient for, or popular with, target audiences.

There are, then, limitations to radio broadcasts (and other mass media activities) as a solution to reach-related problems, but it *is* possible to reach a large segment of even rural audiences through radio broadcasts. By and large, the obstacles to achieving audience attention (including radio distribution, language, time of day, competition from other stations, and poor-quality programming) can be dealt with, although the cost is sometimes high, The major doubt is whether attention so purchased translates into behavior change and nutritional status change.

We can summarize briefly what has been suggested thus far about the reach issue. Face-to-face outreach strategies promise effectiveness, at least on a pilot basis, but may be expensive and logistically difficult if expanded. They show effectiveness but not reach. Radio broadcasts, in contrast, promise reach but have not, up until now, shown the ability to produce nutritional status change. Media broadcasts and outreach from clinics to the homes of potential clients are both strategies for extending the audience for nutrition education beyond the walls of clinics. A third strategy is to expand the number of people who come regularly to a central location where they become an audience for education. Food supplementation programs have been the obvious opportunity for such expansion; and, indeed, next to the haphazard education offered in clinics, they are probably the most common location for nutrition education activity. However, we shall hold off looking at such interventions since they fit best in a discussion of strategies for providing complementary environmental change.

Quality and Systematicness of Education
A fundamental misperception that plagues the design of many educational programs is the confusion between educational channel and educational effectiveness. While no nutrition educator (or any other sort of educator) would admit that the curriculum was less important than putting the channel in operation, that is how most programs in fact operate. Curriculum development may be a side issue. In most projects, minimal funds are spent on prior investigation of the issue being addressed; on the shaping and pretesting of the messages to be offered; on the training, retraining, and supervision of field workers; and on maintenance research

to permit constant adjustment of messages based on audience response. It is true that without reach, effectiveness is irrelevant, but the reverse is no less the case.

While it would be foolish to suggest that none of these educational development activities has gone on in previous projects, two recent nutrition education projects provide a quantum leap with regard to these efforts. One of the projects, the Indonesian Nutrition Education program, relied primarily on village volunteers to carry its messages; the second, the Mass Media and Health Practices project, relied primarily on radio.

Indonesian Nutrition Education. This World Bank–funded program was built on a preexisting base of village volunteers in nutrition (*kaders*) who were already weighing children and giving nutritional advice. The primary activities of the program were to build up the quality and intensity of nutrition education offered by these kaders, and in addition to develop and transmit brief radio programs and posters supporting these activities (Griffiths et al. 1982).

The specific activities undertaken (through the collaboration of Manoff International and the Department of Health in Indonesia) began with approximately nine months of developmental investigation, including preparation and pretesting of radio messages. and continued wth the training of the kaders, usually through a first training course and a refresher course during the year of the program.

The developmental investigation included meetings with community members and leaders and, most important, 330 household interview–case studies. Specially trained interviewer-investigators spent up to two weeks in each village working with ten mothers each. In two- to three-hour sessions, they would explore a variety of relevant educational themes. For example, an interviewer would recommend a trial change in dietary practice such as a new recipe for weaning food or an addition to the mother's diet. The interviewer would then check on the feasibility of the proposed change in dietary practice after a few days of trial by the mother. Guidelines for what interviewers were to learn from each interview were clear but flexible with regard to question strategy. The information so collected was used extensively in the design of educational messages. Radio messages were developed and pretested with a sample of the mothers, and again modifications in language and format were incorporated as a result.

The specific training curriculum for kaders is not extensively described, but it incorporated a two-stage process in which regional leaders were trained and they in turn would train the local kaders. An action poster was given to each mother that allowed her to note her compliance with a particular recommendation from the kader. Apparently, the training served as substantial motivation for the kaders. The kaders who received it reported spending about twice as much time per month in this activity (13 hours versus 7 hours) as did kaders who were not trained. They spent the extra time mostly in supplementing monthly weighings with home visits.

The results of this focused nutrition education effort were impressive. Samples were drawn from the districts receiving the intensive nutrition education (NE) treatment after the program had operated for one year, and from similar control communities visited by nutrition volunteers who had not had the intensive training. There were significant differences in favor of the NE households on many variables including energy consumption and, of most importance, weight-for-age after five months.

None of the families in either the experimental or control communities had significant access to supplemental food. Exposure to radio messages was overall less frequent than had been expected (largely because of dependence on donated broadcast time) and, in any case, spilled over into control areas. The broadcasts could not have produced the experimental group's advantage, although they might have reinforced the kaders' motivation or knowledge, or reinforced for the mother the message she was already receiving from the kader. It is not possible to disentangle the effects of the remaining common elements of the NE strategy, including motivation of the kaders, quantity and quality of advice the kaders gave, action posters, and weighing and use of growth charts.

The Indonesian Nutrition project was essentially a curriculum and volunteer training project. Its success speaks to the value of doing education with care, rather than merely doing education. The essential incremental costs of this add-on project were of two types: the developmental effort and the extra training and kader maintenance activities. The developmental effort was largely a capital cost (although as the project continued beyond one year elements of it needed redoing to keep the activity on track) and could be divided among all recipients in a relatively homogeneous area. The area of the NE project included about 50,000 children and 2,000 kaders. The largest ongoing cost was the training of new kaders and refresher activities for continuing kaders. Obviously, the kader dropout rate was a crucial determinant of ongoing costs. Some cost estimates for this and other projects are provided below.

The major question to be raised about the project is the same as that raised about all outreach programs. High dropout rates among kaders plagued the previous version of this program. While during the experimental year dropout was not a significant problem, whether that will continue to be true in subsequent years or in an expanded program is unknown. The importance of enthusiastic Indonesian leadership and foreign consultants cannot be underestimated in novel programs of this sort. Routine larger-scale programs may suffer without those advantages. Also, the possibility of replication outside Indonesia, where volunteers willing to commit 13 hours per month may be more difficult to find, is an open issue.

Mass Media Health Practices. The second instructional design project was implemented by the Academy for Educational Development (under USAID funding) with the governments of Honduras and The Gambia (Smith et al. 1980). As with the Indonesian project, the most impressive aspect of the Mass Media Health Practices (MMHP) program was the amount of preplanning investigation that went into project and message design. The following describes this work in Honduras.

Based upon an analysis of the medical problem [infant diarrhea] and the communication and instructional requirements of the media to be used, specific investigation topics were established as follows: (1) rural understanding of and response to diarrheal episodes in children under five; (2) general rural child care practices; (3) infant feeding patterns with special emphasis on breast feeding; (4) home-based mixing trials of WHO oral therapy solution; (5) potential sources of bacterial contamination in rural homes; (6) existing distribution systems for commercial medicines; (7) health system outreach; (8) rural media habits and preferences; and (9) rural opinion leadership.

The nine-month investigation used a number of general strategies to collect information on each of these topics: the collection and analysis of existing information (statistical, anthropological, and anecdotal); individual interviews with 175 rural people; 62 focus group interviews with approximately 402 rural individuals; direct observations in 24 rural homes; visits to five rural clinics; plus interviews with pharmacy and rural store owners as well as leading physicians and nurses (Smith et al. 1980, 4).

The investigators report that the results of the developmental investigation were "central to the design decisions...in [the] implementation plan" (p. 4).

The project focused on the treatment of diarrheal episodes and in particular advocated the use of oral rehydration techniques. It incorporated intensive use of radio in a variety of formats, training of local health workers, and education of the professional health community. The curriculum derived from a detailed behavioral analysis of just what steps need to be undertaken in the course of treatment of diarrhea and dehydration. While radio was the central message-delivery method, in both The Gambia and Honduras a significant back-up role was assigned to local workers who served without additional pay. They were the repository of proper mixing instructions for the ORS fluid in both countries, and the source of prepared packets in Honduras. Thus MMHP was not a pure example of a media-only program, just as the Indonesia program extended beyond face-to-face methods.

Results of the program in Honduras and The Gambia indicated widespread self-reported adoption of ORS and other recommended practices. In The Gambia over 50 percent of the target population was aware of the correct mixing instructions and reported using the recommended water, sugar, and salt solution for the last case of diarrhea. Almost no one did so at the outset of the project (Foote el al. 1986). A subsequent implementation of the strategy in Swaziland produced similar results (Hornik and Sankar 1986).

In all three programs, almost everyone in the target audience was exposed to the program messages and a substantial part of the audience learned the recommended behaviors in sufficient detail so that they could perform them effectively (that is, giving ORS, mixing it in a certain way, and administering the right quantity of it) and said they had done it for the most recent episode of diarrhea.

A parallel program was organized in Egypt by the Egyptian government with technical assistance from the John Snow Public Health Group. Along with extended television and radio broadcasts in support of ORS packets, there was an intensive professional education program for the medical community and greatly improved access to the ORS packets themselves through commercial distribution channels. Preliminary evidence suggests not only widespread adoption of ORS, but also a sharp decline in infant mortality (National Control of Diarrheal Dieases Project 1985).

These early programs have been successful and are widely perceived to be so. The MMHP program, now called Communication for Child Survival (or HealthCom), is working with many other countries to improve the communication component of health programs. Other countries, persuaded by these experiences and others, have adapted this approach both to increase the use of ORS and to address other nutrition and health practices. As this communication approach is now becoming routine, some questions will need to be answered.

Only the Egypt studies provide evidence about health benefits; other projects rely on various forms of self-reported compliance with recommended treatments. Future evaluations will need to verify that these changes are not just a reflection of compliant reporting but of efficacious treatment. Also, as these projects move away from being pilot programs that receive special attention and investment, will they continue to be empirically based or will they revert to an easier strategy? Will it be possible to replicate the expensive developmental investigation activity and continual audience response monitoring in subsequent projects? Or can less costly and less time-consuming research still prove useful? Smith (1983) reports on a six-week developmental investigation effort in Ecuador meant to serve as the base for a campaign like that in Honduras. Despite the greatly reduced time frame (and fewer interviews and shorter questionnaire), project planners argued that their level of information was almost as good as what they had had for the Honduras campaign. The realization of this model in Swaziland also relied on more limited precampaign investigations and still showed comparable success.

Second, will it be possible to duplicate the ORS success with other behaviors differently located in both material and value systems of potential beneficiaries? Is ORS an "easy" innovation, open to radio messages in a way that other practice changes will not be? In particular, will it be possible to change infant-feeding practices with similar approaches?

In sum, recent projects have gone a long way toward making the message development process more effective. The resources invested in finding out about the audience complement the energy expended in actually producing and distributing the educational product. The results, at least as reflected in the Indonesian NE project, the Honduran and the Gambian MMHP projects, and the Egyptian ORS program suggest such investments are worthwhile. Nonetheless, the resources required for such message development are considerable; they may be, in absolute terms, well beyond what governments expect to spend for nutrition education. If such resources are to be committed, they will reflect significant policy decisions, including a shift of resources from provision of curative services to preventive programs.

Reinforcement of Messages

The logic favoring the use of many channels reinforcing one another rather than just a single channel for delivery of educational messages is incontrovertible. If the health system, radio and extension workers, posters, and community leaders are all saying the same thing ("Breast-feed" or "Use Oral Rehydration Therapy"), the advantages are unmistakable.

- There are less likely to be contradictory messages in the environment, and thus the appearance of a broad, institutionally accepted norm may be achieved.
- Members of the audience are likely to hear the message from more than one source.
- Each channel, if used optimally, is likely to reinforce the message in a distinct way or serve a different function in the diffusion process.
- Each channel will have access to some members of the audience that other channels may not.

No project planner can help but see the advantages, and indeed many serious nutrition education projects include multiple channels as a matter of course. Some of the projects previously described as emphasizing a particular channel were, in fact, broader. The Indonesian Nutrition Education program complemented nutrition volunteers with radio broadcasts and action posters. The Mass Media Health Practices Project gave local health workers a significant (but different) role in Honduras and The Gambia. In Honduras and in Egypt, project staff allocated a good deal of time effort to working with the health-professional community to gain their acceptance of ORS.

The Brazilian national breast-feeding campaign incorporated education of health professionals with direct outreach to mothers through radio, in-hospital encouragement, health worker talks, and mothers' groups (Jelliffe and Jelliffe 1982). Colombia's Integrated Nutrition Improvement Project has planned or implemented many of the same educational activities. Other examples abound (Zeitlin and Formacion 1981).

Perhaps the Tamil Nadu Nutrition Project (World Bank 1980) goes the furthest, if number of channels is the criterion. Its planning document suggests the use of eight different channels for reaching the target audience directly (community nutrition workers, radio, films, newspapers, wall paintings, posters, flip books, and folk theater), and four additional channels for training field workers (trainers, manuals, new bulletins, and filmstrips). Whether all of these will be used in practice remains to be seen. The traditional folk theater has already been eliminated on grounds of cost (Green 1983). Other projects have used individually distributed flyers, comic books, fotonovelas, arm tapes and weight charts, tape recordings, school instructional materials, television, point-of-sale displays, and group meetings in addition to those already mentioned. Further search would no doubt turn up additional strategies.

However, for all the long lists of potential educational channels, estimates of the efficacy of each channel alone or in combination remains a matter of judgment rather than of empirical evidence. This reflects both the lack of evaluation and the difficulty of disentangling the effects of one channel in a multifaceted operational program.

While the logic favoring more channels over fewer is powerful in the abstract, in practice the logic may break down. Additional channels mean additional costs. Producing materials to be distributed through many channels is likely to affect inversely the quality of materials produced for each channel. Managing multiple distribution systems may tie up so much of a project's energy that it leaves little energy for the production of quality materials. To the extent that one channel depends on the simultaneous operation of a second channel, the possibility of failure increases. Thus the decision to use additional channels is often (or ought to be) a closely calibrated decision balancing what is gained and what is lost. The lack of empirical evidence is painful in this respect. Nonetheless, a logical framework for the analysis of such decisions may be helpful, even if not definitive.

Choice of the mix of channels, at best, reflects experience and judgment about the match between the characteristics of a given channel and the functions that it needs to serve. A list of seven such functions follows. Some of the descriptions for each function repeat comments made elsewhere, and some are merely restatements of commonsense notions. The complete list is presented in the hope that it will serve as a framework in examining the utility of a particular mix of channels. Four elements of the list describe characteristics of a distribution system associated with a channel, and three focus on the content that a channel is capable of delivering.

Accessibility. Some channels are more likely to be seen or heard than others. Restrictions on access reflect inadequacy of the distribution system (television and health workers may not reach out into rural areas; flyers require a distribution agent), the cost to the consumer (radios require expensive batteries; group meetings compete with other demands on time), and the intrinsic characteristics of the channel (newspapers may require some family literacy; flyers may require visual decoding).

Having declared that channels are likely to vary in accessibility, and that a designer needs to be cognizant of such variation, little more of a general nature can be said. Judgment about access to a specific channel will vary with the national context: literacy and batteries may be lacking in one place but not in others; government support for local nutrition workers may give that channel wide access in some countries, although probably not in most. Estimates of how many people are reached by a specific channel, how often, and at what cost to whom, are crucial to the decision to depend on that channel. Such decisions must rely on locally gathered data.

Such estimates should reduce the number of pilot projects whose costs per person reached will never allow widespread expansion. They should also lessen the tendency for a mismatch between target audience and audience actually reached. For example, school nutrition education is often justified on the grounds that children influence their parents and will one day be nutrition decision makers themselves. Advocates argue for the potential of school-based nutrition education but are skeptical about the value of current curricula. They argue that school nutrition education is worth doing well (Van der Vynckt 1983; Valdivia 1983). Nonetheless, the commonness of school programs now seems to outweigh their utility; and at the risk of sounding churlish, one must wonder whether the sheer accessibility of school children does not explain their role as audience.

Similarly, careful balancing of reach and cost may reduce the pressures on program managers to use scarce resources inappropriately. Programs in Zaire (Barnes-Kalunda 1981) and in Costa Rica (Burke et al. 1980) faced major pressures to produce television programs, although their high costs and minimal reach to malnourished populations did not justify them.

Some distinctions between apparent access and realizable access are worth emphasizing. In general, any channel that requires *repeated* physical delivery of materials is at risk of failure. Educational systems that rely on the use of cassette tape recordings may founder on the problem of regular exchange of tapes even if tape recorders are available locally. Stories are legion of posters and flyers sitting in warehouses, unseen by their intended audience. Radio broadcasts may never reach listeners if they are relegated to unpopular times, or if broadcasters fail to comply with schedules.

In general, the choice of a particular mix of channels creates varying demands on a managerial system if access is to be realized. The existence of, or the ability to build, such managerial capacity (whether it be for the supervision and retraining of field workers, for the monitoring and evaluation of a radio system, or for the regular delivery of comic books) must precede the decision to make use of a particular channel.

Repetition and Intensity. A channel that allows a message to be repeated is in most cases to be preferred over one that does not. Neither the practice of complex skills (like the mixing of oral rehydration fluids) nor the acceptance of new norms is likely to result from a single exposure to a message. There are some exceptions ("jobs available — come Monday"), but they are not likely to include most nutrition education themes. The slide-tape to be played for mothers who attend a health clinic irregularly may not achieve repeated exposure. Lectures to groups of mothers by visiting extension workers may face sporadic attendance by both mothers and extension workers. Repeated exposure to messages may be inconsistent and occur only over long intervals.

Radio commercials, played regularly, do offer the promise of frequent and repeated exposure. Television programs, while potentially offering repetition, rarely do so in fact. While most governments initiate broadcasting systems because of their educational potential and promise many educational programs, entertainment and satisfying the demands of urban elites quickly take a primary role. Television hours become too valuable a commodity to be "wasted" on rural education, even if rural communities could be reached.

Still, some "nonrepeating" channels may play a role in an educational program that requires repetition, if they repeat the messages available through other channels. Many countries have mobilized a large number of channels over a relatively short period to create massive practice change. Brazil (Jelliffe and Jelliffe 1982) and Colombia (Valdivia 1983) both chose breast feeding as the subject of massive multichannel campaigns. China has repeatedly made use of national campaigns for various national goals (Chu 1977). Perhaps the Tanzanian campaigns ("Man Is Health" and "Food Is Life") reflect this mobilization strategy most clearly.

The Tanzanian campaigns were massive enterprises, closely linked to the existing political structure. Typically, eighteen months of planning preceded a ten- to twelve-week campaign. Weekly radio broadcasts, widely distributed study guides, and the organization of 75,000 study groups and the training of group leaders for each group were part of the major campaigns. Materials were said to be extensively pretested, and local activities built on the base of preexisting literacy groups and the local cells of the TANU, the single political party of Tanzania. Substantial attention from all levels of government, particularly from President Nyerere, surrounded each campaign.

The 1975 "Food Is Life" campaign was conducted to increase knowledge about nutrition, the use of available foods, and low-cost balanced diets, to eliminate various food taboos, and to encourage better food storage and preservation techniques, better farming methods, and cooperative activities. As many as 1.5 million Tanzanians were estimated to have participated, despite some difficulties with leader training, distribution of printed materials, and access to radio broadcasts (Mahai et al. 1976; Mahai 1976).

No evaluation of the campaign has been published, but evidence from the previous "Man Is Health" campaign suggested substantial short-term effects. The evaluators concluded that, among other health-related changes, over 700,000 latrines were built as the result of campaign activities (Hall and Dodds 1977). Follow-up studies of the extent of subsequent latrine use (or of the maintenance of other new practices) are not available.

Achieving repetitive exposure through the use of multiple channels over a brief period has advantages. It allows the use of some resources that would be unavailable over a longer period; for example, the radio study groups tended to lose members as the campaigns went beyond ten weeks. Explicit public attention by political leaders can be commanded only for brief periods. The sheer intensity of attention may galvanize change that a dribble of messages over a longer period cannot obtain. Mobilization campaigns are less likely than other educational efforts to be lost in the surrounding noise.

On the other hand, mobilization campaigns contain risks. In some contexts they may not be feasible, particularly if there is no preexisting group structure for localizing radio messages and for organizing the immediate realization of recommended behaviors. Budgets for eighteen months of planning, for training large numbers of group leaders, and for coordinating the activities of many institutions may be impossible for some countries. Also, the short-term nature of the Tanzanian campaigns does not allow very much readjustment of messages if problems arise. Once dissipated in the period of the campaign, local energy may be insufficient to encourage the practice of new skills, reinforce changed beliefs and behaviors, and assure their maintenance over time. The dismantling of the educational structure after the campaign may leave no useful way of providing follow-up materials.

Retention. A new nutritional concept or practice has to be retained if it is to be used. Health worker talks, radio broadcasts, and slide-tapes in clinics, when given to nonliterate consumers, all depend on memory as a means of retention. If forgetting or distortion of messages is not to be a great problem, some more permanent memory device is necessary. Flyers, weight charts, posters for home use, newspapers, comic books, and even cassette tapes may be helpful.

There is good reason to believe that such materials are retained over time. Early fears that mothers would lose their childrens' weight and immunization charts turned out to be groundless (Griffiths 1981). Action posters distributed by the Indonesian Nutrition Education Program were to be seen on the walls of many homes well after they were distributed. Higgins and Montague (1972) found that printed materials distributed by the CARE Korean project were still in recipients' hands many months after the campaign ended. In rural homes where little other printed matter is to be found, distributed materials may be treated with special care.

However, visual materials may not serve as memory devices unless they complement other primary channels. Zeitlin and Formacion (1981) cite a study by Fussell and Haaland that is telling. They found that in four of five villages in Nepal no one could interpret a crude poster describing the transmission of tuberculosis, but in the fifth village many could explain what the poster meant. Only in the fifth village had a medical team visited five months before and explained the poster, suggesting that even crude visual materials serve as memory devices, but only if some direct instruction precedes their use.

Spain (1983) found a similar interaction between prior training and ability to decode visual materials in their effects on understanding of a complex flyer. Her study in The Gambia compared women with more and less general decoding skill. For those women with little skill, the direct training they got through radio or from a health worker was a determinant of their ability to decode an oral rehydration flyer. For those women with greater visual skills, their understanding of the flyer was independent of the training they received.

Activity-Passivity. Some educational systems depend on the motivation of potential clients. They make information available but do not actively reach out to the audience. Other systems do not work so passively. The obvious contrast is between professionals in health clinics educating patients who happen to come into the clinic and outreach systems (like Indonesia's Nutrition Education Program) that send volunteers to the homes of community members to encourage their participation.

The activity-passivity factor is as much a reflection of how a channel is used as it is of intrinsic qualities. For example, a radio spot announcement strategy is an active use of the radio channel; it seeks to reach audience members while they listen in an ordinary way to favorite radio programs. In contrast, the broadcast of longer programs on unpopular stations is a passive use of radio, since it depends on the willingness of the audience to seek out information.

In general, it is less complicated and less expensive to manage passive educational systems, but they depend on preexisting motivation of the audience. If people are actively looking for solutions to a given problem, then a reasonably accessible but essentially passive channel may be all that is required. Many parents realize that diarrhea in early childhood is a life-threatening condition, and they anxiously look for solutions (Smith et al. 1980). A relatively passive educational strategy is appropriate in this situation. A weighing program, in a context where parents do not recognize malnutrition, may require much more active efforts for effective delivery.

Combining active and passive channels in a multichannel system may be particularly productive. The Mass Media Health Practices implementation in The Gambia combined an active use of radio with a passive role for village midwives (or other local workers) in the diffusion of ORS. The radio broadcasts provided information encouraging the use of a sugar-salt solution and detailed instruction in its appropriate use. They also mentioned that in each village there was to be found a person with a red flag outside her home who could provide additional information. Each of these persons had been trained in the proper mixing and administration of ORS, and thus served as a secondary source of information for those who had heard and accepted the radio message. Because they were passive educators, the time they would need to spend in teaching was sharply reduced, as was the need for extensive training in outreach methods and for continuing supervision by a central organization.

Accuracy. The more human links a message must pass through before reaching its intended audience, the greater the risk of its being distorted. A nutrition education system that depends on information flowing from originator to supervisor to local trainer to local health worker to client may find that what a client hears is very different from what was intended. Sometimes this poses only a minor danger: pro-breast-feeding messages may be relatively immune from worrisome distortion. On the other hand, home-mixed ORS *is* subject to such distortion, since changes in the proportions of sugar and salt, in the amount of water, or in the amount fed to a child in a given period affects the utility and toxicity of ORS.

Radio broadcasts and other direct channels hold at least a superficial advantage in their potential for accurate delivery of information. Even so, failure to pretest materials sufficiently may risk transmission of information that has a different meaning for sender and receiver. Accuracy of direct transmission may then only be illusory.

Responsiveness. A channel may be responsive in two ways: in its timeliness and in its ability to adjust its messages to individual needs. Each month a new group of mothers becomes interested in messages about child care. A short-lived educational campaign, unless it contrives to leave some residual traces in a community, may be effective with one cohort of mothers but leave subsequent cohorts untouched. Telling in this regard was the follow-up study of the Candelaria project in Colombia, already described. Children born into participating families after the project had terminated were no better off than newborn children in nonparticipating families.

A channel is to be preferred if it allows mothers to seek information when they need it or, at the least, assures a continuous flow of appropriate information until it is substantially accepted in a community. At that point informal diffusion processes may be expected to assure further spread.

Common sense dictates using a channel capable of delivering a timely message. A parallel logic argues for a channel capable of adjusting messages to individual needs. Inevitably, in any presentation of a new recommended practice, there will be doubts to be resolved, further information to be sought, and social support to be gathered. It takes no great logical power to argue that a knowledgeable, skilled, sensitive resource person is ideal in such cicumstances. No radio broadcast is likely to serve that need so well.

Having said this, however, we must now ask about feasibility. Obviously, if a country has the resources to pay for and manage a complete field structure, that is to be preferred. The Tamil Nadu Nutrition Project, for example, planned to hire one local nutrition worker and one assistant for every 1,500 people. Whether this plan (or the expansion of the Indonesian nutrition volunteer program) will be feasible on a large scale, time will tell, although history has not given much ground for optimism. For most countries, however, the issue is whether such responsiveness can be approximated without depending on a vast network of sensitive change agents.

Three mechanisms may provide such approximations. The passive agent, who can be sought out by a person considering change, can resolve doubts and provide social support. Next, even if no paid or formally organized network of agents is available, and only broadcasts provide nutrition education, it is a mistake to believe that individuals make such decisions in isolation. A great deal of social theory and some empirical studies argue that people turn to social networks to support change whether or not such networks are formally organized. It is assumed that decisions to change are taken with careful regard for the expectations of others. A natural corollary is that credible messages about nutrition practice will stimulate the operation of such social support processes. Whether or not those informal social processes will support change or oppose it depends on the circumstances.

A third mechanism for providing responsiveness involves closely following a sample of the audience. This assumes that individual needs are not so particular, and that minimal damage is done if needs are defined and categorized in an aggregate fashion. If that aggregate picture of individual needs then determines what messages are to be sent out, there may be reasonable responsiveness in channels that originate at some distance. An effective monitoring and evaluation program should be able to locate, dynamically, the doubts that exist in an audience and permit effective response. While some individual problems may not be addressed, the largest number should be dealt with.

Independence. An ideal model of nutrition education might involve a smoothly organized set of mutually dependent channels, each taking part of the educational burden in accord with its character. Radio might be relied on for reach and accuracy, face-to-face channels for responsiveness and social support, and printed materials for long-term retention. In such a system, each channel would not be expected to be effective in isolation but only in concert with the others. Such a system might be theoretically ideal, but as a practical matter it is unlikely to be realized. In Indonesia, for example, the radio broadcasts appeared to reach fewer people than expected because of unpopular broadcast times and poor reception in some regions (Zeitlin et al. 1984). In the national Colombian program, coordination between centrally sponsored education (particularly media programs) and local activity was a problem reflecting lack of personnel and institutional stresses (Valdivia 1983).

These examples and many others suggest that channels should be designed to work independently of one another, so that the failure of one will not eliminate all. Inevitable failures of timing, of institutional coordination, and of funding may then reduce the number of sources repeating the same message, but such component failures would not mean system failure. As far as possible, a channel ought to be used with the expectation that no other channel will function adequately.

Ideally a nutrition education system should incorporate a mix of channels that allow maximization of all of these seven characteristics: accessibility, repetition and intensity, retention, activity, accuracy, responsiveness, and independence. While financial limitations and management constraints will make that unlikely, educational system design cognizant of these issues may both make positive outcomes more probable and allow designers a more realistic estimate of what the weaknesses in a particular design are likely to be.

EDUCATION AS COMPLEMENT TO MATERIAL INPUTS

Nutrition education is an anomalous activity. It requires throwing symbols (words or pictures) at malnutrition, a problem that is defined by lack of material resources. Since it provides no new resources, only ideas about organizing available resources, it makes the central assumption that current resources are inefficiently used for desired ends.

In contrast, when education complements newly available resources, its logic may be more persuasive. A change in resources available to a family (through the distribution of subsidized food, the introduction of a new product in local stores, or rapid changes in the prices of staple foods) permits or requires adaptation in dietary practice. In some cases that adaptation will be easy: for example, if the relative prices of two commonly used staple foods were to shift, adjustments in consumption would likely follow shortly. Investment in education to ease that adaptation would have little return. However, in other circumstances education may ease the transition.

In much of Latin America, weaned children are fed only the liquid portion of bean soup. Unfortunately, the solid portion contains much of the nutrition. It is said that mothers do not feed their children beans because beans cause flatulence. Persuading mothers to change this practice has proven to be difficult. An alternative approach is to develop an enzyme "sprinkle" that, when used in small quantities, breaks down the solids, eliminates the flatulence problem, and improves the nutritive value of the food consumed. This solution combines the production and distribution of the "sprinkle" with efforts to convince mothers to make use of it (Rutman 1975).

Food chemists, time and time again, have invented marvelous sprinkles and other synthesized foods only to find that the products do not reach their intended audiences. It would be simplistic and misleading to say that if only they could have joined their products to effective use of communication all would have been well. Problems of product distribution, cost, utility, and acceptability all loom large. On the other hand, if the advantages of the product are not obvious, the likelihood of its acceptance may be increased by an effective education program. The combination of education and material resources has a persuasive logic. Fortunately, there are also a few realized programs based on such a combination for which credible evaluations are available.

Nutrition Education and Food Supplements

A number of evaluated programs combine education with the distribution of subsidized food but do not separate the two components in their evaluations. Four of these are summarized in a review by Gwatkin and his colleagues (1980).

The Imesi project in Nigeria reported greater child growth and lower infant and child mortality in a project area relative to a comparable community, as the result of extensive nutrition education, medical care, and the use of nutritional supplements. A similar project in Jamkhed, India, reported parallel results.

The Narangwal project in India combined nutrition education and supplementation in one of the treatments it offered. When villages with that treatment were compared to control villages, they showed important advantages in growth and mortality. Very similar results were produced in the early 1960s in a five-year experiment in Guatemala by the Institute for Nutrition of Central America and

Panama. Again, nutrition education and supplements had a positive effect on growth and mortality.

These are promising results, but it is impossible to say whether their educational components were necessary for their success. At least one other project summarized in the Gwatkin review (in northern Peru) showed major nutritional changes also, but as the result of nutritional supplements provided without education.

Only one program evaluation attempted to separate the effects of education from those of supplements without education. Gilmore and her associates (1980) report on a post hoc evaluation of a subsidized food program in Morocco run by Catholic Relief Services. They compared children who were beneficiaries of a program before and after an educational component was introduced. The education component was a monthly twenty- to forty-minute class offered at a center where women came to pick up a monthly food supplement. (The supplement amounted to 135 kilograms per family per year, a substantial amount.) The classes were described by the evaluators as dynamic and highly interactive, the result of a major effort to develop a nutrition education capability in Morocco. The subjects included nutrition, health, sanitation, hygiene, and food preparation. Approximately 150,000 families (including mothers, an officially designated beneficiary child, and a sibling) were served at a total of 300 centers. Three monitors per center served twenty-five women each day. The total cost per family was about $103 in 1979. The portion of add-on costs for operating the educational program was only one percent of the total. If administrative and other costs are shared between components, the cost for education amounted to no more than 3 percent of the total.

The reported differences in nutritional status were very large between those children who received both supplements and education in 1978 and their older brothers and sisters who had been enrolled in the supplement-only program three years before. In one comparison, controlling for length of time in the program, among the children who received supplements only, 33 percent were less than 80 percent of weight-for-age standards. In contrast, among their younger siblings enrolled in the feeding-plus-education program in 1978, only 11 percent fell below the 80 percent standard. A parallel comparison between children already in the program and those just entering in 1978 showed similar results.

The evaluators do not believe that the results can be explained by differences in the supplement component of the program or in longer-term secular trends in Morocco. They conclude "an impressive nutritional impact was achieved with the addition of an education program" (p. 6). The evaluation is well considered, and the results appear to be striking. One unresolved anomaly, however, is the apparent failure of the 1975 supplement-only program to have any worthwhile effects on nutritional status. Children who received the supplement but no education in 1975 were more or less comparable to children just entering the program in 1978. One would have expected that an income transfer of this magnitude, estimated to be equivalent to 5 percent to 25 percent of family income, would in itself have had a noticeable effect. Its failure to show any such effect may be seen as additional confirmatory evidence for the conclusion drawn by Cantor and Associates from Figure 7.1 (see p. 109). The underfeeding of young children is not determined by income.

While the results are impressive, there remain issues of great concern, largely to do with the cost and feasibility of expansion. The authors estimate that only 11 percent of all malnourished children in Morocco were reached through this mechanism. The cost of expansion to the entire malnourished population would be high. While mothers do pay a fee (about $6.50 annually), the rest of the cost per family is paid by the government of Morocco ($33) and by international aid programs ($64). If the Moroccan government had to finance the project on its own without international aid and purchase foodstuffs locally, the costs would be even higher. It was estimated to be about $19 million (with $1 million of that contributed by mothers). That would be the equivalent of $126 per family served.

If the program were to reach the entire malnourished population, the total would be $175 million per year (at 1979 prices). The cost per center might also rise as less-accessible portions of the malnourished population were reached. The inflationary effects of such a huge governmental demand for food would affect both the costs of the program and the ability of target families to purchase food besides the ration provided.

This program is probably a special case. In situations where subsidized food is being provided to a population, organized education as a complement to the supplementation may markedly improve the nutritional consequences. However, as a method for reaching entire malnourished populations, it faces obvious financial obstacles. While the add-on costs of education are minimal, the add-on effects are apparently quite large. But, if the $1 educational component can only be effective once the $125 nutrition supplement is delivered, few countries will be willing or able to finance that level of income transfer.

As a final note about this important project, while detailed information about the nature of the educational program is not provided in the evaluation, its authors say that the effort reflects careful planning and execution. There is no reason to believe that many other food supplementation programs that provide education in a much more haphazard way would gain equal success (Anderson 1977).

Social Marketing Projects
Four other projects also complement new resources with education, but they are somewhat distinct from the previously described set. They all can be called *social marketing campaigns* — that is, they make new products available and provide appropriate education, but without subsidizing the new products permanently. The smallest of these was the Yapese coconut campaign.

In Micronesia, a campaign to promote the drinking of green coconut "water" instead of imported and expensive soft drinks was initiated and carried out for two years by the Yap District Health Department (Rody 1978). (The District of Yap is a group of seventeen inhabited islands.) The project used a comic book, in-store posters, and some direct lobbying to encourage stores to stock and people to buy "drinking coconuts." The only newspapers on the island published a photograph of coconuts with a caption that indicated they were the "real thing" and a well-known soft drink the artificial thing. Most young Yapese adults are literate and the slogans soon became popular catch phrases around the district, according to the evaluator. Also a series of cartoons, not originated by the nutrition project, appeared in the paper showing a canned soft drink representing unpopular foreign influence and a coconut character representing Yapese sentiment. Arrangements were made to assure local stores an adequate coconut supply.

As a result of the campaign, most stores on the four main islands began keeping cold coconuts in their refrigerators and selling them for half the price of soft drinks. Several individual stores reported average sales of 1,000 coconuts weekly per store on the main island, even though the total population is less than 4,000. Based on district tax receipts, imports of soft drinks to Yap decreased to less than half their previous level after the campaign (Rody 1978).

Two small projects and one larger one attempted to increase the consumption of soybeans, a food of high nutritional value. Unsurprisingly, given the earlier discussions, the small projects reported signs of success but the larger one was rather less promising. A small-scale program was conducted by Community Systems Foundation (1976) in Colombia and was directed toward educating communities to increase the utilization of soy protein in diets. They used an innovative approach, that of opening a small self-supporting shop, a *tombolita*, which was staffed by local women who prepared and sold soy products like milk and cheese. The women also conducted in-store and in-home education. A survey found that 60 percent of the families in the test city, Villa Rica, had received instruction in soy utilization. A store survey found that of the thirty-seven stores in Villa Rica, seven were selling soy and millet in quantities sufficient to close the average protein gap in the community by 10 percent.

A second small-scale experiment was conducted in two Brazilian villages (Wright et al. 1982). In both villages a brief period of free soybean distribution was followed by a four-month period of availability at a subsidized price. In both villages, groups and individuals were taught how to prepare soybeans and what nutritional advantages could be gained by including them in the diet. Before the campaign, no mothers reported soybean use in their twenty-four-hour recall. At the end of the campaign, about 25 percent of the women in both villages reported soybean consumption in the previous twenty-four hours. (Soybean use had reached a high of 50 percent in one village during the period of free soybean distribution.) It is not known whether this rate of use was inflated because mothers were aware of the investigators' expectations, and whether any use that was achieved was maintained after the subsidies were eliminated. Some doubt with regard to the latter issue comes from the final project reported in this section, the Bolivian soybean utilization project.

The University of North Carolina School of Public Health (n.d.), working with the Bolivian Ministry of Health and USAID sponsorship, mounted an eighteen-month campaign to increase the use of soybeans in rural Bolivia. Soybeans were not previously consumed. The program made use of radio (one fifteen-minute program and six to ten jingles per day) and an extensive program of cooking-method demonstrations in target villages.

At the end of the program, the evaluation suggested that information levels about soybeans were high, that over 80 percent of the population had tried them, and that 45 percent had cooked them at home. However, eighteen months into the campaign, the real nutritional impact remained very small — only 2.5 percent of the sample reported using them in the previous twenty-four hours. The evaluators attributed the failure of the campaign to the complex cooking procedures required, including soaking the beans on the previous day in ash water and boiling them.

Large-scale social marketing programs were also undertaken on behalf of a variety of synthesized foods — most notably Incaparina, an umbrella term for various mixtures of vegetable protein, originally developed by the Institute for Nutrition in Central America and Panama (INCAP). Designed as a low-cost substitute for milk products, it achieved substantial sales in Guatemala, and in related versions in many other countries. Published information does not provide many details about the educational campaigns (or marketing campaigns) that accompanied its commercial distribution, and thus comment must be limited. However, the impact among the malnourished was apparently minimal, largely because the cost of the product placed it beyond their resources even though it was far less costly than milk products (Wise 1980).

This result raises the fundamental question about social marketing programs of the sort reviewed here: Can they be organized to be self-supporting yet still be of benefit to the malnourished population? The Yapese coconut project was, but its audience had sufficient income to purchase soft drinks, and thus was not comparable to the undernourished populations of most concern. The small soybean projects do not provide evidence as to whether they could survive without subsidies or outside organizational help. The Bolivian soybean project did not survive, but financial outlay was less of an issue in that circumstance than was the additional time required for soy preparation. The Incaparina program did survive; enough manufacturing skill went into its preparation to assure its appropriateness, but the unsubsidized costs of commercial preparation put the product beyond the resources of its target audience.

The issue is not educational effectiveness; doing better campaigns for Incaparina-like foods may increase their use and nutritional benefit only minimally. The issue is economic feasibility. A social marketing campaign must market some product, but if the product cost is high, effective marketing may make no nutritional difference. Educational campaigns that enable families to make better use of foods they already consume may suffer less from such constraints.

The several ORS projects described earlier, to the extent that they emphasize the marketing of packets, are also social marketing programs. They face the long-term issue of financing also. If most cases of diarrhea are to be treated with packets, the cost to a government that must distribute them for free may be unacceptable. In Indonesia, for example, the government has decided to allow commercial outlets to sell packets to complement free (but often less accessible) distribution at government clinics. Government-financed media spots recommend both government clinics and commercial outlets as sources for packets.

INCENTIVES FOR EDUCATORS AND CLIENTS

What keeps projects going after the first and novel period? What keeps health workers reaching out and clients coming to clinics? What keeps education, if it is to be delivered at hundreds or thousands or millions of sites, at a high level of quality? The law of entropy is important here: if nothing is done, things tend to fall apart.

The pressures against long-term maintenance of any centralized social service delivery system are large. Those pressures include poor communication within a system, which means that failures are not detected and little is known centrally about clients; lack of funds for transportation, which lessens supervision; and the allegiance of field-workers to their salary-paying bureaucracy, which makes them more responsive to demands from above than to demands from clients.

Educational delivery systems face special problems. When the product to be diffused is education, failure to deliver it adequately may be hard to detect. If food supplements pile up in warehouses, they can be seen; if expected supplements are not obtained, potential recipients may protest vocally. In contrast, poor education is unlikely to leave visible traces or generate loud complaints. Without subtle evaluation, it may remain undetected. This makes it difficult to provide incentives for educational success or remediation in the case of failure. The material rewards for doing face-to-face education well may be small. Psychological rewards — whether the satisfaction of doing a job to the best of one's ability, or the personal gratitude of clients — may be the only incentive. That may work for some educators some of the time, but it may not be enough when a large, long-term, routine program has to be operated.

Clients, like the educators, may be little motivated to participate in nutrition education programs. Mothers, the primary audience, are a group with extraordinary demands on their time. Many projects implicitly assume that only if education would accompany food supplements or health services, or if it comes to them in their own homes, will people sit still for nutrition education (Gilmore et al. 1980). It is not felt that education per se is commonly valued strongly enough to draw an audience on its own. While that assumption may confound client disinterest with poor quality of education, it still may be a reasonable operating assumption.

The problem of creating sufficient incentives over the long run has prompted a number of solutions, both to maintain educational outreach and to encourage client participation. Mass media programs can foster educational outreach; they sharply reduce the need for incentives to make a program effective since they do not depend on motivated field agents. Even in mass media programs, however, some mechanism to maintain the link from field to studio is crucial; without it there is some temptation to reward quality of production without regard for pedagogical effectiveness.

For programs that do not eliminate face-to-face outreach altogether, a variety of approaches to create incentives for field-workers have been implemented. In the Indonesia Nutrition Education project, volunteers were willing to contribute thirteen hours each month, apparently with rewards of a limited sort: social approval by their communities and irregular material rewards (some volunteers received bicycles or rabbits). Apparently volunteerism is widespread in Indonesian communities, and largely nonfinancial rewards may be sufficient. Expansion of this approach past the first year and to other cultures may not be easy.

A second type of incentive is to make the nutrition educator directly respons- ible to the community rather than to the government bureaucracy. If nutrition educators are hired and paid by the ministry, responsiveness to the community may not be a high priority. If the community pays the salary, or at least controls hiring and firing, power over the educational system is effectively transferred. In the agricultural part of this book, we noted a number of programs where extension agents are directly employed by groups of farmers — for example, the Taiwan farmer information system and the Tiv Bams in Nigeria. These programs apparently have greater success that is typical for extension systems (see Chapter 4). Also, traditional curative health systems are directly paid for by their users. The problem with applying this model to nutrition education is that many communities cannot or will not allocate resources to employ a nutrition educator, even when they are willing to do so for agricultural or curative health services.

A third approach, essentially within the social marketing approach, is to provide rewards to educators for achieving behavior change. The traditional midwife may turn out to be a much more effective diffusion agent if she sells an oral rehydration mix packet than if she is given a small salary for undertaking free distribution. Her incentive to make sure that each potential buyer takes full advantage of and is pleased with the ORS solution is strong. The Yapese coconut campaign provided similar incentives for storekeepers (if one can assume that their profit on coconut sales more than balanced losses from depressed soft-drink sales). The Colombian soybean shops begun by Community Systems Foundation were also designed to be self-supporting: the more satisfied buyers of soy products and the more people who knew how to prepare them, the greater the reward for the shopkeeper.

If nutritional benefit can be achieved as the result of introducing a new product, self-supporting educational systems may be feasible. (They may also have negative effects, including a risk that education is designed to maximize sales rather than maximize nutritional benefit; for example, a trusted sales agent may recommend use of an inappropriate product because its profit margin is higher.) However, the applicability of this strategy may be sharply limited. Education for breast feeding or for improving the nutrition of small children, for example, does not seem amenable to such self-supporting approaches. In these areas, with some exceptions (soybeans and enzyme sprinkles were earlier examples), educational strategies are not likely to find a product on which to build a self-financing system.

Clarification of the incentives for the maintenance of individual educational activity and for continued client participation are most crucial to large projects like those in Tamil Nadu and Colombia. These depend on the actions of vast networks of field-workers, whose incentives to provide nutrition education may be uncertain. While the delivery of food supplements and curative services may be supervised straightforwardly and be demanded by clients, educational services are neither easily supervised nor strongly demanded. In that context it may be difficult to ensure that education actually occurs as planned without explicit and directed incentives for educational success.

COSTS AND FINANCING

How much do these projects cost and who pays for them? The costs range from a few cents to more than $100 per family reached. Tanzania put the cost of its "Man Is Health" radio campaign at nine cents per listener; and open-broadcast programs, like those in Sri Lanka and Costa Rica, may have per-listener costs of only a penny or two. The Moroccan feeding programs cost more than $100 per family if the feeding component is seen as an incentive for participation in the educational program. Pilot programs, which involve expensive staff and reach small audiences, may cost even more per person reached.

These cost figures, although they may be in "hard" dollars and cents, tell us little. First, cost estimation methodologies are inconsistent. Cost elements included or excluded from a given estimate will vary from project report to project report. Shared administrative costs, the value of contributed labor and participant time, and the cost of capital and of technical assistance may be added to budgeted outlays of a project or they may be ignored. Without knowing how each of these elements was treated, an observer can make no use of a given estimate. Project reports that provide such information are rare.

The second major concern with raw cost estimates is that they are out of context. A cost estimate not associated with a specific outcome or benefit is essentially meaningless. Without effectiveness criteria, one project's costs cannot be compared to costs for any other project. However, some projects have provided both cost and effectiveness data. Such cost analyses are worth further discussion.

The Moroccan nutrition education program added $1 to $3 to the cost of the food supplementation program already in operation, and apparently produced a decline from about 30 percent to about 10 percent in the proportion of children served who were below 80 percent weight-for-age. If we assume the cost was $2 per family reached (or $1 per child reached if two children were helped in each family), and that about one-fifth (30% − 10%) of all children served were saved from malnutrition under the criterion chosen by the evaluators, the cost per additional child saved was about $5. (The cost of the education plus food supplement would be about $250 per child saved.) A lower criterion of malnutrition (for example, 70 percent weight-for-age) would obviously raise the cost per child saved considerably. A recognition that other children, besides those kept above the 80 percent level, would also have gained some nutritional benefit from the education would lower the cost per child helped.

The Indonesian Nutrition Education project estimated its recurring costs at about $100,000 per year (Griffiths 1983). With 50,000 children in the program, the cost per child was about $2. At eighteen months of age, approximately 17 percent of the children in the Nutrition Education program were below 75 percent weight-for-age. Among comparison children, about 33 percent were below that level (Zeitlin 1984). Thus, about 16 percent (33% − 17%) of the children were saved from such malnutrition, and the cost per case of malnutrition avoided would be about $12.

The Mass Media Health Practices project in Honduras put the in-country cost of operating a parallel program at around $140,000 per year. This includes ministry salaries and the costs of operating the project as well as in-country technical assistance (Shepard and Brenzel 1985). One evaluation report suggested that some 85 percent of the target population, or about 170,000 mothers, heard the ORT messages. Thirty percent reported using the method for the last case, and if these reports can be taken at face value, the cost per adopter was about $2.75 (Foote et al. 1983). An alternative set of calculations, which assume a much smaller target audience, estimated that the cost per episode treated with ORS was $1.10, and the cost per child $1.67 in 1985 dollars, including only in-country expenses. A parallel estimate for The Gambia was $.22 per episode treated and $.44 per child (Shepard and Brenzel 1985).

The Manoff Philippines campaign in Iloilo had 15,000 potential beneficiaries (babies from 6 to 15 months who might potentially have oil added to their weaning food). Nonexperimental project costs were estimated to be about $50,000. About 5 percent of the audience reported adding oil daily (if in minimal amounts). If there were 750 adopting children (5 percent of 15,000), the cost per adopting child would have been about $20 (Zeitlin and Formacion 1981).

Making sensible use of any of these estimates is a difficult business (Jamison et al. 1978). None of the projects counts the value of the participants' time in the educational activity. But a project that takes a person away from other productive tasks (to go to a clinic for a class) has different financial implications from a project that reaches audiences in their homes and takes minimal time from other activities.

Most of the projects for which cost estimates are available have also had large foreign assistance components. A tendency to discount those costs as not representative of what such an operational project would cost is understandable. Nonetheless, if those investments are relevant to the success of a program, they need to be amortized and included in long-term cost estimates. Similarly, start-up costs, including training of personnel and baseline research, may not be treated the same in all projects. If they represent capital expenditures whose benefits will not be played out for a number of years, they also have to be amortized properly. Thus for the Manoff Philippines campaign, future use of available materials would have cost less per person reached than their cost in the pilot year. Unfortunately the cost estimates available come from the early years of projects, and long-term benefits have not been estimated, making the association of costs and benefits problematic.

There is also some tendency to focus on the costs that governments have to pay and ignore other costs. The Indonesian Nutrition Education program relied on the donation of thirteen hours per month by village volunteers (one for every ten families in the program). The monetary value of their labor was not a cost to the government, and the previous estimate of costs for this project ignores this component. However, the volunteer labor represents the largest portion of person-hours spent in the project, and if this cost is left out of cost estimates, it is misleading. The appearance of comparable costs between the Indonesian and Mass Media Health Practices project is tenable only if costs to governments are at issue.

In sum, cost-effectiveness estimates are not easy to put forward with any confidence. Effectiveness criteria vary widely, as do determinations of what is or is not to be included in estimating costs. One could easily imagine cost estimates one-tenth as large or ten times as large as the ones reported above. While more thorough estimates may bring more stability, even those will be ambiguous since they will be estimates of short-term returns on investments with long-term (but unspecified) benefits.

Chapter Nine

Communication in Nutrition: Conclusions

RESTATEMENT OF FINDINGS

At the beginning of this part of the book we asked three questions: What is the potential for educational interventions? Do such interventions as have been evaluated have any worthwhile consequences? And, Is it possible to extend effective programming on a large scale? It is probably an optimistic note that for one of these questions, the second, we can generate a satisfactory and positive answer.

A review of potential areas for educational intervention finds that few nutritional behaviors can be described as unequivocally open or closed to education. Knowledge of the determinants of particular practices is thin, although current research in some of these areas may remedy this situation. However, there is no particular reason to believe that such determinants can be generalized across cultures or other differentiating circumstances.

· Most authors seem to believe that aggregate household nutritional status is largely closed to nonincome intervention and that intrahousehold food distribution and inequity of nutritional status is open to such interventions. That consensus, however, may reflect less valid research than one might like. Nonetheless, most projects seem to act on these assumptions, emphasizing breast feeding, the feeding of weaning-age children, the treatment of diarrhea, special diets for pregnant and lactating women, and improving the balance of meals and sanitary practices. The best evidence for the openness of these behaviors to educational interventions is likely to come from evaluations of those interventions, rather than from basic research on determinants.

Indeed, while the great majority of nutrition education remains unevaluated and is apparently (and probably reasonably) assumed to be ineffective, a few projects show substantial effects on behavior and nutritional status. In Morocco, education together with food supplements produced greater nutritional status change than did supplementation alone. In Micronesia, social marketing of coconut milk as a substitute for imported soft drinks led to widespread behavior change. In Indonesia, nutrition education by village volunteers, supported by radio and action posters, produced a noticeable improvement in nutritional status. Media-based projects in the Philippines, Tanzania, Honduras, The Gambia, Egypt, and Swaziland have reached large audiences who display new knowledge and changed attitudes and report some practice change. For those projects it may be that nutritionally significant change is occurring as well.

However, these successful projects are not representative, nor do they show that nutrition education can be done routinely and effectively on a large scale, when measured against nutritional status. The tension between reaching large audiences, which media-based programs can do, and producing nutritionally significant behavior change, which pilot outreach projects can do, remains the central problem of nutrition education.

The large-scale expansion of face-to-face outreach projects remains fundamentally problematic. Recruiting, training, and supervising the necessary field-workers is likely to be a huge task. Paying them in cash or providing them with sufficient incentives to keep them working effectively over the long haul will be expensive and difficult. Agricultural institutions, with their large budgets and long history of building extension systems, have rarely succeeded in reaching the poorest farmers or in changing their practices (Orivel 1981). Optimism about the probability of the health system's (or a nutrition subdivision's) achieving that end must be limited. Few countries will be able to muster the absolute budgets, the management skill, and the long-haul enthusiasm that will be required. Nonetheless, building on extended health systems, where they do reach the poorly nourished and have a preventive as well as a curative mission, will surely be welcome. Perhaps the only way that face-to-face nutrition education will be realized effectively on a large scale will be if communities take administrative and financial responsibility for such programs on their own, and depend as little as possible on help from outside. If a community is paying for a service, it will take full advantage of it.

It appears that education can bring about change and that the relevant educational concepts are well within the grasp of at least some members of each community. Theoretically, locally operated education is feasible. If limited equipment (for example, weighing scales) and training were available from outside and sought by the community, effective nutrition education might be realized autonomously. The fundamental constraint would be the willingness of and feasibility for a particular community to organize. Some cultures will accept shared communal responsibility with little outside stimulus. Other cultures are less likely to do so.

The alternative route is to rely essentially on mass media programs, complemented when possible by specific face-to-face and other support activities. The central problem of media-based programs is their tendency to become dissociated from what goes on in the field. A radio program takes up the same broadcast time and may sound the same to the urban professional ear, whether or not it is based on any close link with the field. Yet the effectiveness of radio programs, if they are the products of producers and not educators, is likely to be a matter of chance. It is essential that prior investigation, instructional design, pretesting, responses from the audience, and readjustment of messages all be linked.

Stressing instructional design and field research in media-based nutrition education has major implications for cost. Budgeting for field activities and for instructional design, as well as for actual production and the purchase of media time, may not be easily accepted. Absolute budgets directly allocated to nutrition education will be much higher than is customary, even if cost per client reached effectively is likely to be lower. The Mass Media Health Practices program, even without its technical assistance component, cost $125,000 annually, although the cost per self-reported adopter of ORT in Honduras was only $2.50. Yet without these relatively high central costs (for broadcast time, materials preparation, and data collection), effective nutrition education is not likely to be achieved.

Other questions about the usefulness of the mass media remain open. Some argue that the media affect only superficial knowledge or practices, and not behaviors that are more complex or important for an individual (Rogers and Shoemaker 1971). They suggest that the personal face-to-face support of a trusted friend is necessary for change in most circumstances. However, an alternative view may be plausible also. People who are actively seeking solutions for problems will make use of any source that responds to their needs; if they are not anxious to change, face-to-face persuasion will be no more effective than mediated communication. If media-based programs have been ineffective, it does not reflect an intrinsic weakness but the scarcity of programs that have used media well. There is no evidence that sophisticated media-based programs cannot work.

Another objection to mass media programs is a fear that much nutrition education content is too complex to broadcast. People give only fleeting attention to radio, it is said, and cannot learn complex material. It may also be argued that people have sharply varying needs; any attempt to address a heterogeneous population with a single set of broadcasts ignores real differences in prior knowledge, in personal circumstances, and in possibility for change.

Both of these concerns deserve some weight. Nonetheless, there is now a good deal of experience with curriculum development and programming for radio; it suggests that quite complex messages can be broadcast and that a substantial range of the intended audience will be able to take advantage of the information. The Basic Village Education program, which provided agricultural information in Guatemala (Academy for Educational Development, September 1978), the Radio Mathematics project, which taught primary school students (Friend et al. 1980), and the Mass Media Health Practices projects described previously were all successful in teaching complex material via radio to intended audiences.

Despite its potential limitations, media-based education merits a serious look. It may be the only realistic strategy. Any approach that reduces the political, financial, and, most of all, logistical complexities on which projects so often founder is worth a major trial.

Persuasive logic and some empirical evidence suggest that linking nutrition education with other resource changes is a promising approach. The logic is that whenever the old rules do not work optimally, people are likely to be open to new information that allows them to adapt. Supplemental food supplies allow different feeding patterns; education can enable consumers to make optimum choices. Newly available foods or new prices for previously consumed foods may, similarly, allow dietary change. Education can ease the transition.

Another kind of link, also often recommended, is perhaps not so easy to support, although the logic behind suggesting it seems straightforward. (1) The agriculture extension agents are already in the field; it is wasteful to have single-purpose agents. (2) Development is multifaceted; focusing on only one problem risks exacerbating others and is parochial. (3) Therefore, why not build on what extension agents do, and have them become nutrition agents?

Nonetheless, as a practical matter, linkages with other agencies' activities are not likely to work. (1) Agricultural extension agents rarely get to the poorest farmers, and by definition ignore landless laborers, yet those two groups are among the most malnourished, and women are rarely a direct audience for them. (2) Extension agents in more sophisticated systems, like the Training and Visit System, are fully loaded with specific agricultural tasks and would resist taking on roles as multipurpose agents. While backyard gardens and the raising of small animals for protein may fall more directly in their purview, it may be unrealistic to expect agents to take on these tasks. In any case, such practices are rarely high priority for nutrition education programs. As appealing as linkage with another, richer sector's activities may be, its promise for success is not great.

IMPLICATIONS

Finally, what are the implications of all this for people concerned with nutritional status and nutrition education? First, how should a national planner considering strategies for combatting malnutrition look on nutrition education? The first thing is to stop looking at nutrition education in the traditional way — as a minor activity involving a few posters and irregular clinic-based advising, run out of a basement office in the Ministry of Health with no budget or status. If nutrition education is to be worthwhile at all, significant goals of behavior change for large audiences need to be adopted, and budgets and personnel commensurate with those tasks need to be allocated. A planner needs to choose a serious purpose and then ask whether nutrition education is a competitive strategy for accomplishing that goal. He or she ought not to be asking what improvements can be achieved within current minimum budgets. The answer is likely to be very little. In general, if it is politically unrealistic to expect larger budgets for nutrition education, then it is going to be unrealistic to expect worthwhile consequences.

The next issue is to ask whether nutrition education, no matter how effectively implemented, is likely to affect a particular nutritional concern. In some cases, diagnostic information will eliminate education as a useful strategy. If withdrawing the breast during an episode of diarrhea is rare in a particular culture, or occurs because of sick childrens' lack of appetite and despite mothers' attempts to feed them, it is not likely to be an appropriate target for nutrition education.

If economic circumstances preclude practice change, or if a recommended change is likely to have a minimal effect on nutritional status, there may be little point in addressing it with education. Water boiling, both because of the demands it makes for fuel and time and because it may have little effect on infection in the face of so many other environmental sources of infection, is an example on both counts.

If lack of knowledge remains a possible cause of poor practice in a given culture, next come questions about what educational strategies are feasible in a particular context. What field structures are in place and reaching the target audience? Is there a saturated network of distribution points for products? How far do agents who might take part in an active educational network reach? What incentives are likely to encourage effective delivery of education? Can backup training and supervision be implemented? Is there a network of agents who would be able to be part of a passive educational system, even if expecting effective and active outreach is unrealistic? What proportion of the audience can be reached by radio, given language and ownership issues? What level of community responsibility for nutritional improvement is likely to be activated? Is there a reasonable possibility of local and autonomous management of education-based change?

Given the experience summarized in this book, the answers to these questions are likely to lead away from face-to-face active outreach education systems. This is particularly likely to be the case if one has to build a network from scratch or depend on people whose salaries are paid by other bureaucracies, and if communities cannot be expected to take long-term financial and administrative responsibility for local activity.

Prior experience will lead either to some skepticism about the viability of edcuational strategies altogether because they are so difficult to implement, or to the construction of media-based education systems. They promise audience reach, logistic feasibility, and at least a reasonable potential for success. Such systems probably need to assume that people are open to change and are looking for solutions to problems they currently or could easily recognize. The problem for media-based systems is to find appropriate educational messages, reflecting solutions that fit with the lives and preferences of audiences, and then to communicate them clearly so that they permit action. The point is not to develop cosmetic broadcasts that give only the appearance of action, but to tie media messages to knowledge of audiences. Broadcasts linked to concommitant resource or environmental change are particularly promising, and such links may be crucial for some areas of practice change.

Part Four

Conclusions

Chapter Ten

Doing Communication for Development

In the first chapter of this book, there was tempered optimism about the future of communication for development. Yet the fact is that few of the programs in agriculture and nutrition described in subsequent chapters have produced much change. How is the apparent contradiction to be resolved? The answer lies in the explanation for failure that appears most credible now.

At the start we offered three broad explanations for that result: (1) Information is no solution for a lack of resources; (2) Audiences for information programs are unresponsive even when such information might help; and (3) Information programs have not worked because they have not been done appropriately. Certainly all three explanations are correct some of the time. Yet, of the three, the explanation that most demands our attention is the third, which focuses on the doing of projects. While it has been immensely difficult to realize mass information and education campaigns, it is possible to do them better. And it is this possibility that gives cause for optimism.

To say that the problem is in the doing of projects is not to say that the answer is better "doers," or managers; the managers who lead projects are often able. Rather, the problem is that mass information projects as they are commonly designed are fundamentally unmanageable. The solution is to design programs that are possible to manage and that are realistic, given the context of a particular less-developed country.

Here we shall try to make this position explicit. First, we summarize evidence from previous chapters that supports the argument that the design of information programs is a central problem. Next, we present a prescriptive section: How might manageable, effective information programs be designed. Finally, we will ask, Given how programs have evolved in the past, what likelihood is there that in the future more projects will achieve their desired goals?

COMPARING EXPLANATIONS FOR PROJECT INEFFECTIVENESS

If, at the beginning of our discussion, we had had to guess which explanation would be the centerpiece of the final chapter, we would have chosen not the third but the first of the three, that information is no solution, given that the essential problem is lack of resources. In Chapter 2, it was called theory failure, and if any theme dominates current writing about information and development it is this one. It reflected a strong counterreaction to the psychological theories of the 1950s and 1960s that placed much of the blame for failure to change on individuals: on farmers and mothers who maintained traditional farming and health practices despite contrary advice from the modern sector. The psychological theories of David McClelland (need for achievement), Everett Hagen (entrepreneurship), and Daniel Lerner (empathic personality) all suggested that the slow pace of development reflected the failure of societies to generate people with appropriate prodevelopment personalities.

However, these "individual blame" theories found less acceptance in the atmosphere of heightened social criticism of the late 1960s and early 1970s. Other views that were less prone to blame the poor for their poverty became prevalent. There was a strong argument (and some evidence) that people failed to heed advice from outside not because of personal fatalism or traditionalism but because they were structurally bound to current practice.

Theodore Schultz argued that farmers in developing countries were highly responsive to economic rewards and that failure to adopt an innovation occurred when the potential rewards did not counterbalance the risks. Jeremiah O'Sullivan found that farmers in the Guatemalan highlands who rejected no- or low-cost innovations (like compost piles and seed spacing recommendations) did so reasonably. He could find no evidence that farmers who did adopt such agronomist-recommended innovations were more productive than those who did not. Carlos Benito found that farmers in Mexico who did not adopt a Plan Puebla–recommended planting package did so with good economic justification. While the package did produce greater yields and profits, it also required more labor. And that labor, it turned out, could be sold elsewhere at a higher return than if it had been used for farming.

Surely such structural factors, like lack of access to credit to purchase fertilizer or too little income to purchase an adequate diet, set upper limits on how much change is possible. However, knowing that failure to innovate is *sometimes* economically explained is not evidence that it can *always* be explained economically. There is counterevidence that supports the notion that worthwhile change is possible, given fixed resources. It is clear that some groups, given equal resources, make more of their circumstances than others. The Amish in Pennsylvania, Japanese farmers in Brazil, and kibbutz farmers in Israel have all been able to make more of their farms than others around them, and those differences cannot be explained by capital alone. Marlaine Lockheed, Dean Jamison, and Lawrence Lau (1980) bring together studies supporting the effects of farmer schooling on productivity. When newer technologies were available, farmers with more than four years of schooling produced about 10 percent more than their neighbors with no education but equal resources. These studies only reinforce what any informal or formal study of farming communities suggests: that some farmers outperform others consistently, regardless of resources.

It is also likely that nutritional status is not completely determined by income. While household income and household nutrient consumption are found to be highly correlated, there often remains the possibility of improvement even without additional income. Jere Behrman and Barbara Wolfe found that in Nicaragua additional income did not go primarily to nutritional improvement even in families whose current diets were inadequate. Sidney Cantor and his coauthors (1973) studied the feeding of weaning-age children in Tamil Nadu in India. They found that the inadequate feeding of young children persisted among families whose income should have provided adequate nutrition to every family member.

All this is not to be taken as evidence that some farmers are bad and others good or that some families are nutritionally concerned and others are uncaring. Nor is it to suggest that agricultural output and nutritional status are not primarily determined by resource availability. Rather, it makes the point that characteristics not related to current resource availability can affect current practice. For some people in some circumstances, information about how best to organize available resources may promise improved agricultural productivity and nutritional status. This book points to common circumstances when current practice is not ideal — that is, when practice does not reflect the best way to organize current resources to maximize agricultural benefit and family nutritional status.

In agriculture this may occur when changes in the "rules" come at a rapid pace: with new credit arrangements, new markets, changed prices for supplies or products, or newly available technologies. Under those circumstances, altered practice would permit a higher return, even respecting resource availability.

In nutrition the potential for improvement may also reflect opportunities created by a changing environment: varying food prices or food availability and improved technologies (like oral rehydration therapy for treatment of dehydration). The largest benefit at the lowest cost may involve programs for particularly vulnerable groups like small children and pregnant or lactating women.

If there is substantial potential for information in development, why isn't it being realized? Must we return to individual blame theories? Are some people simply more innovative than others, more psychologically willing or intellectually able to adapt as useful information from the modern sector flows toward them? Or is the problem that potentially useful information doesn't do much flowing? Do the potential beneficiaries of information not have the opportunity to be innovative because they do not see the useful information in accessible form?

Sorting out explanations is difficult, but if one must choose either audience stubbornness or poor information availability as a primary explanation, the second is to be preferred. From each of the following perspectives it is the better operating assumption.

Available studies suggest that conventional information distribution channels are typically weak. They may reach a small proportion of the potential audience and they carry information that is either dated or unresponsive to the needs of the audience. Agricultural extension agents are too few, have too little research and logistical support, and are too rarely rewarded for successful work with farmers. Health and nutrition education is most often a burdensome additional activity for the predominantly curative health services; ambitious outreach programs atrophy with time.

Time after time, a close look at conventional face-to-face educational programs finds little match between the sort of education that is supposed to be occurring and what actually occurs. There are too few staff incentives, and there is too little organizational support to maintain, over the long term and on a large scale, effective face-to-face communication in most contexts. Outside of schools, where organizational support can be substantial, face-to-face education may have requirements that are unrealistic. There are exceptions, of course. Short-term campaigns, with concentrated political support, may be feasible and effective for a limited set of information goals. Also, information services that are purchased by the audience directly rather than entirely supplied by the government may serve well. However, neither short-term campaigns nor user-purchased information services are the norm in developing countries.

The failure of conventional programs to reach their audiences supports the explanation that nonoptimum practice reflects a poor flow of information and not an unwillingness of audiences to respond. Additional support for the "poor flow" argument comes from smaller-scale projects that do operate effectively, if only for the short term and in pilot areas. Some projects in agriculture and nutrition provide solid evidence that information programs *can* affect farm output and nutritional practice and status. These projects are not always evidence about effective ways of investing in information (their expansion to a mass audience may not be logistically feasible), but they are evidence that investments in information can effect desired outcomes. If done well, information programs make a difference. The question is how to do them well.

Finally, a preference for the explanation that points to poor information delivery rather than audience unresponsiveness reflects a policy requisite. Explanations that suggest that a shift in policy may assist in the effectiveness of information services are preferred because they offer a potential point of intervention. Individual unwillingness, to the extent that it is the operating explanation of current practice, is effectively beyond the reach of sectoral planners. In contrast, the shape of information delivery services, while constrained by political and financial forces, is potentially amenable to policy change. On these grounds, acceptance of the poor delivery system explanation, if at all tenable, is defensible.

To summarize, there is reason to believe that current resources will allow changed practice in particular circumstances; there is reason to believe that individual unresponsiveness is not a sufficient explanation for current practice; there is reason to believe, in contrast, that current information programs rarely provide *adequate* information flows, but that effective provision of information has made a difference. The remaining question is how to do information for development well, over the long term and on a large scale.

PRESCRIPTIONS FOR DOING INFORMATION FOR DEVELOPMENT WELL

So much for the diagnosis. The potential and the problems are easy enough to describe. The difficult issue is how to do information programs well. With some coaxing seven prescriptions emerge from the earlier material.

Financial and Managerial Feasibility
Is there sufficient money to operate the system if it reaches its full audience? Will it be possible to manage the system, given available personnel and the complexity of the administrative structure? Is it possible to develop an incentive structure that will reward successful work, over time? A conventional face-to-face system rarely will permit a yes to any of these questions. Budgets suffice only to reach a portion of the intended audience; managers find the supervision of isolated field agents to be a difficult task; and the agents have few rewards for doing the job as the manual says it must be done.

Responsiveness
Is there a mechanism that assures that the messages in the information channels are responsive to farmers' needs? Is there anything worth communicating? Is there potential for positive change in a particular context? Will recommended changes prove productive for adopters at an acceptable risk? Are they presented in a form respectful of the worldview of the beneficiary? Will they solve a problem the audience sees as needing solution? Are they locally adapted? Do they respond to the diverse needs of a heterogeneous audience? Are they presented through a channel that is accessible to the audience? Information programs serving large, distant, dispersed audiences require an information-gathering mechanism that provides guidance about the messages that are useful, about the channels that will reach the audience, and about the nature of the audience, and that does so over time.

Message Development
The other side of responsiveness is making effective use of knowledge about the audience once it is available. Knowing what is useful does not assure that messages reach audiences in a form that is accessible. Is there time and talent within the operating structure of an information system to make materials that are pedagogically effective? Are distribution channels sufficiently free of distortion so that what is heard reflects what was meant to be heard?

Integration with Other Institutions
The effectiveness of an information service is constrained by its links with other institutions working in its sector. The information service must respond to changes in agricultural credit availability and technology and to the travel schedules of vaccination vans. Consistency in the action of all relevant institutions

makes a great deal of common sense and, for some information programs, may be their only route to success. At the same time it may be difficult to achieve, given the relative autonomy and distinct reporting lines common enough in bureaucracies. Exacerbating this isolation (for example, by locating the information service for a given sector such as agriculture in a cross-ministerial information authority) ought to be done with full recognition of the possible loss in intrasectoral institutional integration.

Support in the Process of Change
Changes in practice, whether in agriculture or nutrition, are rarely simple; they may involve multiple actions repeated over time; they may demand concomitant changes in other aspects of family life; they may involve perseverence in a new practice when the rewards for first attempts are small or delayed; they may involve challenging more or less strong social norms. The strongest theoretical argument favoring the presence of a flesh-and-blood change-agent focuses on the potential for providing a channel for resolving doubts and for obtaining reinforcement for hesitant steps down the path to change. Making cohesive groups the target of field agent activity has a similar justification. If groups change together then individuals can find local support.

The incorporation of a field agent and group support makes sense. The lack of specific supporting evidence is not grounds for counterargument. Nonetheless, as a practical matter, developing effective face-to-face field agents and organized group support rarely has proved feasible. While admitting that such a support network would be good if it were feasible, one may still ask if it is crucial.

To some degree the focus on field agents and group support is the reflection of earlier psychological theories of development and their focus on the reluctant-to-change, fatalistic traditionalist: if people are reluctant changers they require face-to-face support to convince them to act against their natures. We have assumed, contrarily, that people are anxious to solve problems of agricultural productivity or of health and nutritional status and that they are actively seeking ways to do so. The cajoling of the trusted agent is not so obviously central, given that operating assumption.

Also, there is an implicit assumption in the organized-support model that without it the individual members of the audience are isolated in their consideration of new practices: if outsiders do not organize a support network it will not exist. Yet most literature on social change argues in the opposite direction. Suggested change stimulates the operation of "natural" reference group networks, whether outsiders encourage it or not. Individual decisions to adopt a new practice are rarely taken in isolation; rather, they are the product of interaction with preexisting social networks.

Organizd support may be an ideal, but it may be unachievable. Practically, if a mass information program is to proceed at all, it can rarely involve an active face-to-face outreach channel. Nonetheless, even if there is some skepticism about the need for the cajoling function, there can be little question of the need to know and respond to the doubts and concerns of the audience. To the extent that those doubts and concerns are widely shared, a constantly operating feedback system involving a sample of farmers and a production system capable of turning feedback into responsive messages may serve as a partial substitute for the organized support system.

Patience

No information program is going to be a panacea for all development problems. Few programs will affect all members of their intended audience; most will take years, rather than months, to realize worthwhile goals. As politically difficult as this may be, little of lasting value is likely to be achieved without choosing targets judiciously, without substantial commitments of funds and without extended work over time. Some innovations are so extraordinarily advantageous and so risk-free that they will spread rapidly with minimal information efforts. But then most of these would have diffused of their own accord without any public investment in information flows. Most changes in practice are not of this sort, however.

Some proposed innovations are of small absolute benefit to their adopters but of great value in the aggregate: any single dose of oral rehydration solution has only a small probability of saving a child's life — but as a community practice, it may save many children who would otherwise die each year; a new seed variety may produce only a few percent gain in output for any one farmer but, accumulated across a nation's farmers, may mean a large total gain in food supply.

Innovations may be complex, they may produce small absolute rewards, they may depend on the slow evolution of complementary institutions, they may depend on the activation of natural social networks. Although many members of the audience may be reached directly with information, the success of an information campaign may still depend on natural social diffusion processes in a community. One may find that knowledge diffuses rapidly, but change in actual practice may occur slowly.

Noninstantaneous response ought not be a matter of frustration but a recognition of realistic expectations. Patience — and the resources to maintain a program for a sufficient time and at a sufficient level of energy to match realistic estimates of how fast change will occur — should be incorporated in the plans for any information program.

Political Attractiveness

To the extent that an information program calls on a public budget to achieve its ends, it must build a supportive constituency and avoid creating political enemies. Having developmentally "good" objectives may not be sufficient. Political supporters must be able to derive direct benefits; they ought to be able to earn political visibility and credit with their own supporters. On the other hand, challenging entrenched groups in the design of an information program is a risky path. Even if it made technical sense to abandon a salaried agricultural field agent system to channel money to an alternative information service, it would usually make political nonsense. Political cost-benefit ratios must affect the design of an information service, particularly if a program is not to remain an isolated international showpiece but to become part of the national budget over time.

IMPLICATIONS FOR THE DESIGN OF INFORMATION PROGRAMS

If these are some general prescriptions, what are the concrete implications for design of information services?

Media-based Rather Than Active Face-to-face Programs

Face-to-face programs are to be preferred, theoretically, over the media-based, which are, in contrast, financially and managerially possible. They have a "star" quality that may lead to political support. They may be managed closely and thus it becomes possible to coordinate with other institutions and to obtain extended materials development. They increase the probability of a match between intended messages and messages actually received.

Investments in Audience Monitoring and Program Research.

Media projects tend, powerfully, toward isolation from their audiences. All information services need the ability to understand what practices may be affected by information and how current practice is related to the rest of people's lives. They must be able to monitor change in response to an ongoing campaign or other outside factors. They need to be able to test the appropriateness of messages before they are incorporated in an information program. Most of all, an information service needs a structure that not only allows for the use of such information but absolutely depends on it. The built-in incentives for integration of field information gathering and materials production must guarantee their coordination.

The studies reported in this volume suggest that a major problem of existing information systems is the development of messages worth communicating, rather than the unwillingness of audiences to accept good advice. The transfer of resources from extension activities (which in any case reach only a small portion of the audience) to intelligence gathering can be justified. The same extension agents, who are often ineffectual diffusers of information, may turn out to be invaluable as gatherers of information. With a constant presence in the field and charged with sampling audience members in a systematic way, they can develop information that can hold message producers to the realities of the field.

Incorporation of Passive Channels

A distinction has been drawn between active outreach channels, where it is the responsibility of the field agent to reach out physically to potential beneficiaries, and passive outreach channels, which serve as local repositories of information but which must be sought out by beneficiaries. The contrast is between paid or volunteer agents who are required to go out to find and weigh babies and give nutritional advice to mothers, and agents who are available in their homes to those who wish to seek them out for prepared oral rehydration salts packages or for mixing instructions for the home-mixed sugar-salt solution.

In both cases, the goal is to provide the direct support for change so often advised. Passive channels, which rely on the willingness of beneficiaries to seek out help, fit with an assumption that audiences are actively seeking solutions to problems. At the same time, the requirement for limited training and minimal supervision avoids the overwhelming logistical concerns of organizing, supervising, and maintaining an active outreach system. Passive agents (which may include health posts or pharmacies and local offices of agricultural institutions as well as specifically recruited agents) also may serve as distribution points for printed materials, which are often necessary as memory devices to supplement ephemeral radio broadcasts.

Links to a Substantive Ministry

The costs of developing separate information services for agriculture, nutrition and health, and other development sectors are high, given scarce resources and scarce talent. The temptation to develop an integrated communication-for-development service to serve as the technical arm across development sectors is great and justifiable. Still, in the long run, it is likely to be a false economy. The tendency for information programs to become isolated from their audiences and from sectorally relevant institutions is large. Any bureaucratic distance between information producers and the institutions that are substantively responsible for programs in a sector will increase that tendency. There may be short-term costs paid in quality of production by tying an information service to a budget-short ministry; nonetheless, if that service can be more easily integrated into the operating chain of that ministry, those costs are likely to be bearable. Integration will encourage responsiveness to sectoral concerns; it will offer some hope of complementing information activities with the concrete resource providing activities in the sector; it will provide a home and establish a call on a sectoral budget without the unrealistic need to assume that cross-ministerial collaboration with and budget subsidization of a central communication and development service will go on indefinitely.

In sum, an information service with the most promise depends on a mass medium as its central delivery mechanism, incorporates field agents as passive channels, is linked with a substantive ministry, and spends much of its energy and budget gathering and analyzing information in order to respond systematically to the heterogeneous needs of its audience. Returning to earlier themes, it addresses important targets that justify the expense of a slow and intense materials production process and require patience toward the pace of consequential change.

THE CHANCES OF REALIZING THE RECOMMENDED MODEL

How likely is it that the path outlined here will be followed? It is, admittedly, a politically difficult path. On the one hand, the recommended prescription is not altogether dissimilar to what is being done currently (radio for development is nearly universal) and is close to some of the projects now operating on a short-term or pilot basis. Nonetheless its serious adoption requires a major reordering of budget and personnel allocations.

In health and nutrition education, few countries now invest in more than marginal ways. Curative services receive the lion's share of most budgets, and health education offices remain in the corner of ministry basements. Building an information service with substantial materials-development capacity and, more burdensome, a significant field staff for information gathering and analysis is not consistent with current conceptions. A decision to move in that direction often implies a struggle with the existing medical establishment. Trading radio time for hospital beds may seem an unattractive exchange.

In agriculture there is a longer-standing commitment to, and investment in, extension services. However, the existing conventional system (even if dissatisfaction with it is widespread) will not be readily turned into the radically different system proposed here. Even if the jobs of existing agents were protected by asking them to take on different functions, such change is likely to be perceived as threatening. Existing systems may not work efficiently for their intended beneficiaries, but they may work quite well for their employees.

There is another problem: the argument for a media-based system is by no means unchallengeable. Agriculturalists, in particular, even if they recognize the failings of conventional systems, find it difficult to imagine extension without active agent outreach and demonstration. Success in some short-term projects in nutrition and health and equivocal success in agriculture, which is the best the state of the art offers, are underwhelming grounds for arguing that this is a sure path to large-scale, long-term success. There is a mixture of conceptual reasonableness and empirical evidence in the approach to information provision advocated here. Some might prefer less reasonableness and more evidence.

Others would add to these concerns about the viability of the proposed strategy a more general political qualification. These approaches argue for spending additional monies to benefit the poor, usually rural, populations of developing countries. If new information programs end up as isolated broadcasting projects with no field structure, it may reflect less a technical disbelief in their efficacy than a political unwillingness to commit the funds. Engaging in an extended discussion of the best ways to provide information for development smacks of technocratic naïveté to those critics. Their first concern is to understand why programs of this sort are rarely realized. Political naïveté and technocratism are terrible accusations to level against a development scholar or planner (even if self-directed). There are a few responses.

There are many countries whose commitment to benefiting the rural poor is real enough, if limited. Whether that reflects a loyalty to a political constituency, a belief in the long-term nation-building benefits of investment in the poor, or an ideological commitment to benefiting the least advantaged need not be argued.

Also, media-based projects may not always require new monies, only a reallocation of existing budgets. A program proposed at a moment of dissatisfaction with current arrangements, involving actions (like radio broadcasts) that promise political visibility for their proponents and drawing international funding for some capital costs and technical assistance, may turn out to be politically attractive.

What then is the prediction for the next decade? Will it be possible to talk about realized and successful information programs in agriculture and nutrition? There seems little reason to doubt that the state of the art will become increasingly sophisticated. The trend in the design of information services describes a continuing upward path. Knowledge about how to do this activity well both grows and diffuses. International agencies (U.S. Agency for International Development, the World Bank, the UN agencies, and national development agencies of many nations) are clearly committed to continued investment in developing and implementing such systems. On these grounds, the number of evaluated models for media-based information systems is likely to increase. More countries will have had first-hand experience with the approach. They will have had an opportunity to choose this information model after some direct experience with it.

A first prediction, then, is that many more countries will have experimented with sophisticated communication and education programs, either as pilot programs or as short term efforts. A second prediction is that many of those countries will be pleased with the results (and the plaudits associated with addressing serious problems in a publicly observable way), and will extend the programs. A third prediction, one less satisfying than the previous two, is that many of those extended programs will lack the resources they need to maintain all elements of the sophisticated model. They will find it easy to reduce or eliminate audience research and intensive materials testing, find themselves relying on donated and less desirable media time, and allow links with the actions of others within and without the ministry to attenuate. Those shortfalls seem likely to be exaggerated in the agriculture sector where the demands for a quite complex curriculum adjusted to regional needs are great. The health and nutrition sector may fare better in this regard. In both cases larger countries, and/or countries which can expect international aid over the long term, will find the absolute development costs more acceptable than others.

A final prediction, or perhaps merely a hope, is that one or more of these large scale implementations will work in an unequivocal way. It will be possible, then, to report evaluation results which establish that worthwhile agricultural productivity or nutritional status improvements are produced by feasible information programs operating on a large scale and over time. Current studies suggest but do not establish this. Unequivocal evidence may both speed the adoption of the sophisticated model, and, by clarifying what it requires, enable practitioners to muster the resources needed to realize it and maintain each of its elements.

Bibliography

Academy for Educational Development. *The Basic Village Education Project — Guatemala: Final Report*. Washington, D.C.: AED, September 1978.

————. *Masagana 99: Philippines—Project Profile*. Washington, D.C.: Clearinghouse on Development Communication, October 1978.

————. *Mass Media and Health Practices: Project Implementation*. Washington, D.C.: AED, June 1982.

Agrawal, Binod C. *Satellite Instructional Television Experiment: Television Comes to Village — An Evaluation of SITE*. Bangalore, India: Indian Space Research Organisation, 1978.

Allen, G. R. *Agricultural Marketing Policies*. Oxford: Basil Blackwell, 1959.

————. "Short-term Variations in Retailing Margins on Fruits in East Paskistan." *Farm Economist* 9, no. 6 (1959): 259–66.

Anderson, C. Arnold. "Effective Education for Agriculture." In Philip Foster and James R. Sheffield, eds., *Education and Rural Development*. London: Evans Brothers Limited, 1973.

Anderson, M. A. "CARE Preschool Nutrition Project: Phase II Report." Unpublished report from CARE, New York, August 1977.

Ascroft, Joseph, et al. *Extension and the Forgotten Farmer: First Report of a Field Experiment*. Bulletin No. 37, Department of Sciences, Wageningen: Wageningen Agricultural University, 1973.

————, and Gleason, Gary. *Communication Support and Integrated Rural Development in Ghana*. Paper prepared for the 30th International Conference on Communication, Human Evolution, and Development of the International Communication Association, Acapulco, May 1980.

Ashby, Jacqueline, et al. *The Economics of Education and Communications System Strategies for Agricultural Development*. Palo Alto: EDUTEL Communications and Development, Inc., 1978.

Austin, James E., et al. *Annotated Directory of Nutrition Programs in Developing Countries*. Cambridge, Mass.: Harvard Institute for International Development, 1978.

Axinn, George H., and Thorat, Sudhakar. *Modernizing World Agriculture: A Comparative Study of Agricultural Extension Education Systems*. New York: Praeger Publishers, 1972.

Balderston, Judith B., et al. *Malnourished Children of the Rural Poor: The Web of Food, Health, Education, Fertility, and Agricultural Production*. Boston: Auburn House Publishing, 1981.

Bammi, Vivek. *The Content of Agricultural Broadcasting in Two Indian States*. M.A. thesis,

University of Pennsylvania, Philadelphia, 1983.

Barnes-Kalunda, Shirley. *Consultant Report for Zaire (February 23–March 17, 1981): Evaluation of the Mass Media Component of AID's Nutrition Planning Project in Zaire.* Newton, Mass.: International Nutrition Communication Service, 1981.

Beaton, G. H., and Ghassemi, H. *Supplementary Feeding Programmes for Young Children in Developing Countries.* Report prepared for UNICEF and the ACC Subcommittee on Nutrition of the United Nations, October 1979.

Behrman, Jere. *Supply Response in Underdeveloped Agriculture: A Case Study of Four Major Annual Crops in Thailand, 1937–1963.* Amsterdam: North Holland Publishing Co., 1968.

———. *The Relevance of Traditional Economic Theory for Understanding Peasant Behavior: A Case Study of Rice Supply Response in Thailand, 1940–1963.* Discussion Paper No. 37. Philadelphia: Economic Research Services Unit, Department of Economics, University of Pennsylvania, 1967.

———, and B. Wolfe. "More Evidence on Nutritional Demand: Income Seems Overrated and Women's Schooling Underemphasized." *Journal of Development Economics*, 14: 105–28 (January/February 1984).

Benito, Carlos A. "Peasants' Response to Modernization Projects in *Minifundia* Economies." *American Journal of Agricultural Economics* 58, no. 2 (May 1976).

Benor, Daniel, and Harrison, James Q. *Agricultural Extension: The Training and Visit System.* Washington, D.C.: World Bank, 1977.

Berg, Alan. *Malnourished People: A Policy View.* Poverty and Basic Needs Series. Washington, D.C.: World Bank, 1981.

Bosley, B. "Nutrition Education." In *Nutrition in Preventive Medicine*, eds. G. H. Beaton and J. M. Bengoa. Geneva: World Health Organization, 1976.

Boyce, James K., and Evenson, Robert E. *Agricultural Research and Extension Programs.* New York: Agricultural Development Council, 1975.

Brumberg, Stephan F. "Colombia: A Multimedia Rural Education Program." In Manzoor Ahmed and Philip H. Coombs, eds., *Education for Rural Development: Case Studies for Planners.* New York: Praeger Publishers, 1975.

Burke, Richard; Hornik, R. C.; Manoff, R. K.; and Cooke, T. M. *Consultant Report for Costa Rica.* Newton, Mass.: International Nutrition Communication Service, 1980.

CARE. *Breaking the Communications Barrier: A Report of Results.* New Delhi, India: Thomson Press Limited, 1973.

Cantor and Associates. *The Tamil Nadu Nutrition Study.* Vol. 1. Haverford, Pa: S. M. Cantor Associates Inc., 1973.

Cassirer, Henry R. "Radio in an African Context: A Description of Senegal's Pilot Project." In Peter L. Spain, et al., eds., *Radio for Education and Development: Case Studies.* Vol. 1. Washington, D.C.: World Bank, 1977.

Chaudhri, D. P. *Education, Innovations, and Agricultural Development.* London: Croom Helm, Ltd., 1979.

Chen, L., and Scrimshaw, N., eds. *Diarrhea and Malnutrition: Interactions, Mechanisms, and Interventions.* New York: Plenum Press, 1983.

Chu, Godwin C. *Radical Change Through Communication in Mao's China.* Honolulu: University of Hawaii Press, 1977.

Clearinghouse on Development Communication. *Health Education Radio Dramas: Sri Lanka.* Washington, D.C.: Clearinghouse on Development Communication, 1980.

————. *Nutrition Advertising Campaign: Tunisia.* Washington, D.C.: Clearinghouse on Development Communication, 1979.

Coleman, W. F., and Opoku, A. A. "Rural Radio Forum Project in Ghana." *An African Experiment in Radio Forums for Rural Development: Ghana, 1964–1965.* Paris: UNESCO, 1968.

Committee 10 of International Union of Nutritional Sciences Workshop Report. "Rethinking Food and Nutrition Education Under Changing Socio-Economic Conditions." *Food and Nutrition Bulletin* 2, no. 2 (April 1980): 23–28.

Community Systems Foundation. *AID First-Year Progress Report: Community Experiments in the Reduction of Malnourishment in Colombia.* Ann Arbor, Michigan: Community Systems Foundation, June 1976.

————. *AID Second-Year Progress Report: Community Experiments in the Reduction of Malnourishment in Colombia.* AID, June 1976.

Contreras, E. "Brazil and Guatemala: Communication, Rural Modernity, and Structural Constraints." In E. McAnany, ed., *Communications in the Rural Third World.* New York: Praeger Publishers, 1980.

Cooke, T. M., and Romweber, S. T. *Radio, Advertising Techniques, and Nutrition Education: A Summary of a Field Experiment in the Philippines and Nicaragua.* New York: Manoff International Inc., December 1977.

Coombs, Philip H., and Ahmed, Manzoor. *Attacking Rural Poverty: How Nonformal Education Can Help.* Baltimore: Johns Hopkins University Press, 1974.

Cronbach, L., and Furby, L. "How Should We Measure Change — Or Should We?" *Psychological Bulletin* 74 (1970): 68–80.

Drake, William D., et al. *The Promotora Program in Candelaria, Part I: A Colombian Attempt to Control Malnutrition and Disease, 1968–1974. Part II: A Revisitation Two Years After Program End.* Washington, D.C.: USAID Office of Nutrition, 1980.

ECA-FAO Joint Agriculture Division. *A Comparative Analysis of Agricultural Extension Systems of Eight East Asian and African Countries — With Suggested Guidelines for Improvement.* Addis Ababa: ECA-FAO, 1971.

Esman, Milton J. "Popular Participation and Feedback Systems in Rural Development." In Robert H. Crawford and William B. Ward, eds., *Communication Strategies for Rural Development.* Proceedings of the Cornell-CIAT International Symposium. Ithaca: Cornell University, 1974.

Evenson, Robert, and Jha, Davanatha. "The Contribution of Agricultural Research Systems to Agricultural Production in India." *Indian Journal of Agricultural Economics* 28, no. 4 (October–December 1973): 212–230.

————, and Kislev, Yoav. "Investment in Agricultural Research and Extension: A Survey of International Data." *Economic Development and Cultural Change* 23, no. 2 (April 1975): 507–24.

————. *Agricultural Research and Productivity.* New Haven: Yale University Press, 1975.

Fagen, Richard. *The Transformation of Political Culture in Cuba.* Stanford, Calif.: Stanford University Press, 1969.

Farquhar, John, et al. "Communication for Health: Unselling Heart Disease." *Journal of*

Communication 25, no. 3 (Summer 1975): 114–26

Feder, Gershon, and Slade, Roger. *Impact of Agricultural Extension: A Case Study of the Training and Visit System in Haryana, India.* Washington, D.C.: World Bank, 1985.

Feder, Gershon; Just, R.; and Silberman, D. *Adoption of Agricultural Innovations in Developing Countries: A Survey.* Staff Working Paper No. 444. Washington, D.C.: World Bank, 1981.

Fisher, J.D., et al. *Agricultural Extension Training: A Course Manual for Training Programs.* Nairobi, Kenya: USAID, Rural Development Division, 1968. (Rpt. Information Resources Division/PDER, April 1970).

Food and Agriculture Organization. *Handbook on Human Nutritional Requirements.* FAO Nutritional Series No. 28, WHO Monograph Series No. 61. Rome, 1974.

Foote, Dennis, et al. *The Mass Media and Health Practices Evaluation in Honduras: The Final Report of the Major Findings.* Menlo Park, C.A.: Applied Communication Technology, 1985.

Foote, Dennis, et al. *The Mass Media and Health Practices Evaluation in The Gambia: The Final Report of the Major Findings.* Menlo Park, C.A.: Applied Communication Technology, 1985.

Foote, Dennis, et al. *The Mass Media and Health Practices Evaluation in Honduras: Findings from the First Year.* Stanford; Calif.: Institute for Communication Research, 1983.

Friend, J; Searle, B; and Suppes, P. *Radio Mathematics in Nicaragua.* Stanford, Calif.: Institute for Mathematical Studies in the Social Sciences, 1980.

Gilmore, Judith W., et al. *Morocco: Aid and Nutrition Education.* AID Project Impact Evaluation Report No. 8. Washington, D.C.: USAID, 1980.

Graham, Jack, and Paige, Donald. "Radio Reaches Rural Teachers in Nepal — But Do They Have the Energy to Turn It On?" *Development Communication Report* 33 (March 1981): 1, 5–6.

Green, James. Personal communication, January 1983.

Griffiths, Marcia. *Growth Monitoring of Preschool Children: Practical Considerations for Primary Health Care Projects.* (Primary Health Care Issues, Series I, No. 3). Washington, D.C.: American Public Health Association, October 1981.

———. Personal communication, 1983.

———; Manoff, R. K.; Cooke, T. M.; and Zeitlin, M. *Mothers Speak and Nutrition Educators Listen: Formative Evaluation for a Nutrition Communications Project.* 2 vols. New York: Manoff International, Inc., 1980.

Gwatkin, Davidson R., et al. *Can Health and Nutrition Interventions Make a Difference?* Monograph No. 13. Washington, D.C.: Overseas Development Council, 1980.

Hagen, Everett. *On the Theory of Social Change.* Homewood, Ill.: Dorsey Press, 1962.

Hall, Budd L., and Dodds, Tony. "Voices for Development: The Tanzanian National Radio Study Campaigns." in P. Spain, D. Jamison, E. McAnany, eds., *Radio for Education and Development: Case Study.* Washington: The World Bank, 1977.

Hayami, Yujiro, and Ruttan, Vernon W. *Agricultural Development: An International Perspective.* Baltimore: Johns Hopkins Press, 1971.

Herdt, Robert W. "Resource Productivity in Indian Agriculture." *American Journal of Agricultural Economics* 53, no. 3 (August 1971).

Higgins, Margot, and Montague, Joel. "Nutrition Education Through the Mass Media in Korea." *Journal of Nutrition Education* 4, no. 2 (Spring 1972): 58–61.

Hornik, Robert; Sankar, Pamela; Huntington, Dale; Matsebula, Gladys; Mndzebele, Alfred, and Magongo, Bogani. *Communication for Diarrheal Disease Control: Swaziland Program Evaluation, 1984–1985*. Philadelphia: Annenberg School of Communications, University of Pennsylvania, 1986.

Hornik, Robert, et al. *The Role of Communication in Education*. Stanford; Calif.: Stanford University, Institute for Communication Research, 1978.

Hudson, Heather, and Parker, Edwin. "Medical Communication in Alaska by Satellite." *New England Journal of Medicine* 289 (December 20, 1973): 1351–56.

Huffman, Wallace E. "Assessing Returns to Agricultural Extensionism." *Amercian Journal of Agricultural Economics* 60, no. 5 (December 1978): 969–75.

Hyman, Herbert H.; Levine, Gene; and Wright, Charles R. *Inducing Social Change in Developing Communities: An International Survey of Expert Advice*. Geneva: United Nations Research Institute for Social Development, 1967.

Indian Institute of Mass Communication. *Agro-Information Flow at the Village Level*. New Delhi, 1968.

Inkeles, Alex, and Smith, David H. *Becoming Modern: Individual Change in Six Developing Countries*. Cambridge, Mass.: Harvard University Press, 1974.

"Interview with Daniel Benor, An." *Development Communication Report* 22 (April 1978).

Israel, Ron, et al., eds. *Maternal and Infant Nutrition Reviews: A Guide to the Literature*. Newton, Mass.: International Nutrition Communication Service, n.d.

Jamison, D.: Klees, S.; and Wells, S. *The Costs of Educational Media*. Beverly Hills, Calif.: Sage Publications, 1978.

Jamison, Dean T., and Lau, Lawrence J. *Farmer Education and Farm Efficiency*. Baltimore: Johns Hopkins University Press, 1982.

————, and McAnany, Emile G. *Radio for Education and Development*. Beverly Hills, Calif.: Sage Publications, 1978.

Jelliffe, Derrick B., and Jelliffe, E. F. Patrice. *Consultant Report for Brazil (March 21–31, 1982): An Assessment of the Brazilian National Breast-Feeding Promotion Campaign*. Washington, D.C.: International Nutrition Communication Service, 1982.

Jenkins, Janet. "Mass Media for Health Education." IEC Broadsheets on Distance Learning, No. 18. Nottingham; Eng.: Russell Press Ltd., 1983.

Katz, Elihu, and Lazarsfeld, Paul F. *Personal Influence: The Part Played by People in the Flow of Mass Communications*. New York: Free Press, 1955.

Kidd, David W. *Factors Affecting Farmers' Response to Extension in Western Nigeria*. East Lansing: Michigan State University, 1968.

Klonglan, Gerald E. *Radio Listening Groups in Malawi, Africa*. Ames: Iowa State University, Department of Sociology and Anthropology, 1967.

Knudsen, Odin K. *Economics of Supplemental Feeding of Malnourished Children: Leakages, Costs, and Benefits*. World Bank Staff Working Paper No. 451. Washington, D.C.: World Bank, 1981.

————, and Scandizzo, Pasquale L. *Nutrition and Food Needs in Developing Countries*. World Bank Staff Working Paper No. 328. Washington, D.C.: World Bank, 1979.

Krishna, Raj. "Agricultural Price Policy and Economic Development." In Herman Southworth and Bruce Johnston, eds., *Agricultural Development and Economic Growth.* Ithaca: Cornell University Press, 1967. Pp. 467–540.

Lazarsfeld, Paul, and Merton, Robert. "Mass Communication, Popular Taste, and Organized Social Action." In L. Bryson, ed., *The Communication of Ideas.* New York: Institute of Religious and Social Studies, 1948.

Lee, Chin-Chuan. *Media Imperialism Reconsidered.* Beverly Hills, Calif.: Sage Publications, 1980.

Lele, Uma J. "Market Integration: A Study of Sorghum Prices in Western India." *Journal of Farm Economics* 49 (February 1967): 147–59.

Lerner, Daniel. *The Passing of Traditional Society.* Glencoe, Ill.: Free Press, 1958.

Leslie, Joanne. "Evaluating Nutrition-Education Projects: Getting the Message and Acting on It." *Development Communication Report* 20 (September 1977).

―――. "Evaluation of Mass Media for Health and Nutrition Education." In *Educational Broadcasting International* VII. No. 3 (September 1978).

Lionberger, Herbert F., and Chang, H. C. *Farm Information for Modernizing Agriculture: The Taiwan System.* New York: Praeger Publishers, 1970.

Lockheed, Marlaine E.; Jamison, Dean T.; and Lau, Lawrence J. "Farmer Education and Farm Efficiency: A Survey." *Economic Development and Cultural Change* 29, no. 1 (October 1980).

Mahai, B. A. P. "Communication Constraints and How They Were Overcome in the 'Chakula Ni Uhai' Campaign of 1975 in Tanzania." Paper delivered at the International Workshop on Communication Constraints, December 1976.

―――, et al. "The Second Follow-up Formative Evaluation Report of the 'Food Is Life' Campaign (June 12–July 21, 1978)." Unpublished paper for the Institute of Adult Education, Research and Planning Department, August 1978.

Manoff, Richard K. *Consultant Report for Brazil, Volume II (March 21–31, 1982): An Assessment of the Communications Component of the Brazilian National Breast-Feeding Program.* Washington, D.C.: International Nutrition Communication Service, 1982.

Manoff International Inc. *Project Description: Nutrition Education and Behavior Change Component: Indonesian Nutrition Improvement Program.* New York: Manoff International, 1983.

―――. *A Summary Report on the Mass Media Nutrition Education Project in Ecuador.* Washington, D.C.: Manoff International, 1976.

Martorell, Reynaldo. Personal communication, 1984.

―――; Habicht, J. P.; and Klein, R. A. "Anthropometric Indicators of Changes in Nutritional Status in Malnourished Populations." In B. Underwood, ed., *Methodologies for Human Population Studies in Nutrition Related to Health.* Washington, D.C.: National Institutes of Health, Publication No. 82–2462, 1982.

Mathur, J. C. *Adult Education for Farmers in a Developing Society.* New Delhi: Indian Adult Education Association, 1972.

―――, and Neurath, P. *An Indian Experiment in Farm Radio Forums.* Paris: UNESCO, 1959.

Maunder, Addison H. *Agricultural Extension: A Reference Manual.* Rome: FAO, 1972.

Mayo, John K., et al. *Development Radio for Nepal: Report of the Radio Feasibility Study Team.*

Stanford Calif.: Institute for Communication Research, Stanford University, 1975.

―――. *Educational Reform with Television: The El Salvador Experience.* Stanford, Calif.: Stanford University Press, 1976.

McAnany, Emile G. *Communications in the Rural Third World: The Role of Information in Development.* New York: Praeger Publishers, 1980.

McClelland, David. *The Achieving Society.* New York: Van Nostrand, 1961.

McDermott, J. K. "Extension Institutions." In Melvin G. Blase, ed., *Institutions in Agricultural Development.* Ames: Iowa State University Press, 1971.

McDowell, Jeffrey. "Comments on Market Information Issues." Unpublished manuscript, n.d.

―――, et al. "The Institutional Functioning of Agricultural Radio and Its Constraints in India and The Gambia." Unpublished manuscript, 1985.

McDivitt, Judith A. "Communication and Agricultural Innovation Under Structural Constraints." M.A. thesis, University of Pennsylvania, Philadelphia, 1981.

Melmed, Arthur, et al. "Everyman's University in Israel: The First Two Years." In H. Perraton, ed., *Alternative Routes to Formal Education.* Baltimore: Johns Hopkins University Press, 1982.

Merton, Robert. *Social Theory and Social Structure.* Glencoe Ill.: Free Press, 1957.

Morgan, Robert M., et al. *Evaluación de Sistemas de Communicación Educativa.* Bogota: Acción Cultural Popular, 1980.

Moris, Jon. *Reforming Agricultural Extension and Research Services in Africa.* London: ODI Agricultural Administration Network Discussion Paper 11, 1983.

Morss, Elliott R., et al. *Strategies for Small-Farmer Development: An Empirical Study of Rural Development Projects in The Gambia, Ghana, Kenya, Lesotho, Nigeria, Bolivia, Colombia, Mexico, Paraguay, and Peru.* 2 vols. Washington, D.C.: Westview Press, 1976.

Mosher, Arthur T. *Creating a Progressive Rural Structure: To Serve a Modern Agriculture.* New York: Agricultural Development Council, Inc., 1969.

―――. *Thinking About Rural Development.* New York: Agricultural Development Council, Inc., 1976.

―――. *An Introduction to Agricultural Extension.* New York: Agricultural Development Council, Inc., 1978.

National Control of Diarrheal Diseases Project. *Fact Sheet.* Cairo, Egypt: NCDDP and John Snow, Incorporated. June 1985.

Nelson, Ralph E., and Kazungu, David K. *An Evaluation of the USAID Extension Saturation Project in Uganda.* Morgantown: West Virginia University, 1973.

―――, and Phelps, E. "Investment in Humans: Technology Diffusion and Economic Growth." *Amercian Economic Review* 56 (May 1966): 69–75.

Nesman, Edgar G.; Rich, Thomas A.; and Green, Sara E. *Individual, Family and Village Literacy in Development.* Tampa: University of South Florida Press, 1980.

Nichter, Mark, and Nichter, Mimi. *An Anthropological Approach to Nutrition Education.* Washington, D.C.: International Nutrition Communication Service, 1981.

Orivel, François. *The Impact of Agricultural Extension Services: A Review of the Literature.* Washington, D.C.: World Bank, 1981.

O'Sullivan, J. "Guatemala: Marginality and Information in the Western Highlands." In

Emile McAnany, ed., *Communications in the Rural Third World*. New York: Praeger Publishers, 1980.

Patel, A. U., and Ekpere, J. A. "Characteristics and Radio Listening Behaviour of Farmers and Impact on Knowledge of Agricultural Innovations." *Agricultural Administration* 5 (1978): 83–90.

Pelto, Gretel H. "Anthropological Contributions to Nutrition Education Research." *Journal of Nutrition Education* 13, no. 1 (Supplement, 1981): S2–S8.

Perraton, Hilary. *Alternative Routes to Formal Education*. Baltimore: Johns Hopkins University Press, 1982.

———; Jamison, Dean; and Orivel, François. "Mass Media for Agricultural Extension in Malawi." In Hilary Perraton, ed., *Basic Education and Agricultural Extension, Costs, Effects, and Alternatives*. Washington: World Bank, 1983.

Pielemeier, Nancy. "The Relationship of Mother's Nutrition Knowledge to Child-Feeding Practices and Child Nutritional Status in Lesotho." Unpublished doctoral dissertation, Johns Hopkins University, 1983.

Post, James. Personal communication, March 1983.

Ramadasmurthy, V., et al. "Nutrition Education and SITE Telecasts." *International Journal of Health Education* 21 (1978): 168–73.

Rasmuson, Mark. "Three Media Strategies Used in Nutrition Education." *Development Communication Report* 20 (September 1977).

Reutlinger, Schlomo, and Selowsky, Marcelo. *Malnutrition and Poverty: Magnitude and Policy Options*. Baltimore: Johns Hopkins University Press, 1976.

Rice, E. B. *Extension in the Andes*. Cambridge, Mass.: MIT Press, 1974.

Rody, Nancy. "Things Go Better with Coconuts: Program Strategies in Micronesia." *Journal of Nutrition Education* 10, no. 1 (January–March 1978): 19–22.

Rogers, Everett M. *Diffusion of Innovations*. 3rd ed. New York: Free Press, 1983.

———; Eveland, J.; and Bean, Alden S. *Extending the Agricultural Extension Model*. Stanford, Calif.: Institute for Communication Research, Stanford University, 1976.

———, and Svenning, Lynne. *Modernization Among Peasants: The Impact of Communication*. New York: Holt, Rinehart & Winston, 1969.

———, and Shoemaker, F. Floyd. *Communication of Innovations: A Cross-Cultural Approach*. 2nd. ed. New York: Free Press, 1971.

Roling, Niels, et al. "The Diffusion of Innovations and the Issue of Equity in Rural Development." *Communication Research* 3, no. 2 (April 1976).

Roy, Prodipto; Waisanen, F. B.; and Rogers, Everett M. *The Impact of Communication on Rural Development: An Investigation in Costa Rica and India*. Paris: UNESCO, 1969.

Rundfunk und Fernseh and Africa Asian Bureau. *Rural Radio in Indonesia: Investigations into Possibilities for Expansion and an Evaluation of the German Rural Radio Advisory Project*. Bonn: Federal Ministry for Economic Cooperation, n.d.

Rutman, Max. Personal communication, 1975.

Ruttan, Vernon W. "Agricultural Products and Factor Markets." *Economic Development and Cultural Change* 17, no. 4 (1969).

Sanghvi, Tina. Personal communication, 1983.

Schramm, Wilbur. *Big Media, Little Media.* Beverly Hills, Calif.: Sage Publications, 1977.

————. *ITV in American Samoa — After Nine Years.* Stanford, Calif.: Institute for Communication Research, 1973.

————. *Mass Media and National Development.* Stanford, Calif: Stanford University Press, 1964.

————, et al. *The New Media: Memo to Educational Planners.* Paris: UNESCO–IIEP, 1967.

Schuh, G. Edward, and Tollini, Helio. *Costs and Benefits of Agricultural Research: The State of the Arts.* Washington D.C.: World Bank, 1979.

Schultz, Theodore W. *Transforming Traditional Agriculture.* New Haven: Yale University Press, 1964.

————. "The Education of Farm People: An Economic Perspective." In Philip Foster and James R. Sheffield, eds., *Education and Rural Development.* London: Evans Brothers Limited, 1973.

————. "The Value of the Ability to Deal with Disequilibria." *Journal of Economic Literature* 13, no. 3 (September 1975): 827–46.

Scrimshaw, Nevin S. "A Look at the Incaparina Experience in Guatemala: The Background and History of Incaparina." *Food and Nutrition Bulletin* 2, no. 2 (April 1980). Tokyo: United Nations University.

Scrimshaw, Susan C. M. "Infant Mortality and Behavior in the Regulation of Family Size." *Population and Development Review* 4, no. 3 (1978): 383–403.

Selowsky, Marcelo. "Nutrition, Health, and Education: The Economic Significance of Complementarities at Early Age." *Journal of Development Economics* 9 (1981): 331–46.

Shepard, Donald, and Brenzel, Logan. *Cost-Effectiveness of the Mass Media and Health Practice Projects.* Menlo Park, C.A.: Applied Communication Technology, 1985.

Shingi, Prakash, and Mody, Bela. "The Communication Effects Gap." *Communication Research* 3, no. 2 (April 1976).

Shore, L. "Mass Media for Development: A Reexamination of Access, Exposure, and Impact." In Emile McAnany, ed., *Communications in the Rural Third World: The Role of Information in Development,* New York: Praeger Publishers, 1980.

Smith, William A. *Dr. Hakim: A New Voice in the Village (Radio Nutrition Education in Tunisia).* Washington, D.C.: Academy for Educational Development, 1979.

————. Personal communication, 1983.

————, et al. *Mass Media and Health Practices Implementation: Honduras Implementation Plan.* Washington, D.C.: Academy for Educational Development, 1980.

Spain, Sikandra. *Factors Affecting Pictoral Comprehension in Non-Literates: Results of a Survey in The Gambia, West Africa.* M.A. thesis, Annenberg School of Communications, University of Pennsylvania, Philadelphia, 1983.

Stockley, Trevor L. *Assistance to Rural Broadcasting: Afghanistan.* Rome: FAO, 1977.

Suchman, Edward A. *Evaluative Research.* New York: Russell Sage Foundation, 1967.

Sweeney, William O. *Using Radio for Primary Health Care.* Primary Health Care Issues, Series 1, No. 1. Washington, D.C.: American Public Health Association, 1982.

Toquero, Zenaida, et al. "Marketable Surplus Functions for a Subsistence Crop: Rice in the

Philippines." *American Journal of Agricultural Economics* 57 (November 1975): 705–9.

U.S. Agency for International Development (USAID). *AID's Responsibilities in Nutrition.* Washington, D.C.: USAID, 1977.

Valdivia, Margaret. Personal communication, 1983.

Van der Vynckt, Susan. Personal communication, 1983.

Van Esterik, Penny, and Greiner, Ted. "Breast Feeding and Women's Work: Constraints and Opportunities." Studies in Family Planning: Breast-feeding Program *Policy and Research Issues* 12, no. 4 (April 1981): 184–97.

Vemury, Merlyn. *Rural Food Habits in Six Developing Countries: A CARE Study on Environmental, Social, and Cultural Influence on Food Consumption Patterns.* New York: CARE, 1981.

Viravaidhya, Khun Vina, et al. *Impact of Age-Weight Charts Maintained in the Home and Nutrition Education on Nutritional Status of Infants and Pre-School Children.* Unpublished manuscript, 1981.

Welch, Finis. "Education in Production." *Journal of Political Economy* 78, no. 1 (1970): 35–59.

Wharton, Clifton R., Jr. "Education and Agricultural Growth: The Role of Education in Early-Stage Agriculture." In C. Arnold Anderson and Mary Jean Bowman, eds., *Education and Economic Development.* Chicago: Aldine, 1965.

White, Robert A. "Mass Communications and the Popular Promotion Strategy of Rural Development in Honduras." In Peter L. Spain et al., eds., *Radio for Education and Development,* vol. 2. Washingon, D.C.: World Bank, 1977. Pp. 200–60.

"Why Are Soviet Babies Dying?" *Wall Street Journal* 30:1, 1983.

Winikoff, Beverly, and Baer, Edward C. "The Obstetrician's Opportunity: Translating 'Breast Is Best' from Theory to Practice." *Amercian Journal of Obstetrics and Gynecology* 138, no. 1 (September 1980): 105–17.

Wise, Robert P. "The Case of Incaparina in Guatemala." *Food and Nutrition Bulletin* 2, no. 2 (April 1980). UN University World Hunger Programme. Tokyo: United Nations University.

World Bank. *Tamil Nadu Nutrition Project: Implementation Volume.* Washington, D.C.: World Bank Population Health and Nutrition Department, 1980.

———. *World Development Report, 1979.* Washington, D.C.: 1979.

———. *World Development Report, 1980.* Washington, D.C.: 1980.

Wright, Maria da Gloria Miotto, et al. "Approaches for Increasing Soybean Use by Low-Income Brazilian Families." *Journal of Nutrition Education* 14, no. 3 (September 1982).

Zeitlin, Marian F. Personal communication, 1984.

———, and Formacion, Candelaria S. *Study II: Nutrition Education.* Boston: Oelgeschlager, Gunn, and Hain, 1981.

———; Griffiths, M.; Manoff, R. K.; and Cooke, T. *Household Evaluation, Nutrition Communication, and Behavior Change Component: Indonesian Nutritional Development Program,* vol. 4. Report to the Department of Health, Republic of Indonesia. New York: Manoff International, 1984.

Index

Academy for Educational Development (AED)
    Guatemala, 76–78, 150
    Philippines, 75
ACPH. *See* Honduras
ACPO. *See* Colombia
Afghanistan
    radio agriculture program, 70, 73–74
Africa. *See also* ECA–FAO.
    extension activities, 51, 54
    farm projects in East, 53
    language problems, 124
    radio schools, 90
Agrawal, Binod, 75, 84, 86
Ahmed, Manzoor, 47–51, 54, 61–62, 64, 67,
    70, 84–85
Alaska, Two-way radio project, 9
Allen, G.R., 41
Amish in Pennsylvania, 156
Anderson, M.A., 31, 140
Ascroft, Joseph, 56
Ashby, Jacqueline, 44
Asia, radio schools, 90
Audience Reach, 18–19, 31, 50–52, 56–61,
    117–125
Austin, James E., 116, 121
Axinn, George H., 43–44, 50, 55, 60, 69

Baer, Edward C., 104
Balderston, Judith, 110–111
Bammi, Vivek, 72
Bangladesh
    consumption survey, 100
    nutrition behavior, 102–103
    weaning, 108
Barnes-Kalunda, Shirley, 132
Basic Village Education program (BVE). *See*
    Guatemala
Bean, Alden, 50, 67

Behrman, Jere, 16, 40–41, 100, 157
Benito, Carlos, 64, 156
Benor, Daniel, 43, 52, 65–66, 69, 85
Berg, Alan, 97, 101, 111
Bolivia
    extension activities, 50
    Ministry of Health, 141
    potato project, 63
    soybean use project, 141–142
Boyce, James K., 44, 48, 50, 52
Brazil
    breastfeeding campaign, 104–105, 130,
        133
    extension activities, 50
    Japanese farmers, 156
    MEB (Movimento de Educacao de Base), 84
    radio and nutrition, 124
    soybean distribution, 141
Breastfeeding, 102–107
Brenzel, Logan, 146
British Open University, 9, 21
Broadcasting, Agricultural, 73–78.
    See also Channels
Brumberg, Stephan F., 81–82
Burke, Richard, 122, 132

Candelaria Project. *See* Colombia
Cantor, Sidney and Associates, 108–110, 140,
    157
CARE
    India Nutrition Program, 122
    Korea Nutrition Program, 122, 134
    Vemury Survey, 102, 114
Cassirer, Henry R., 11
Catholic Relief Services, 139
Chang, H.C., 60, 62–63, 70
Channels
    accuracy, 135–136

Channels (*cont.*)
  activity-passivity, 134–135
  comparison of mass media and face-to-face,
    91–92, 122, 130–137, 149–152
  face-to-face, 87–89, 149, 158. *See also*
    Extension Activities.
  repetition and intensity, 132–134
  retention, 134
Chaudri, D.P., 31–32
Chen, L., 112
China, National Campaigns, 133
Chu, Godwin C., 19, 133
Clearinghouse on Development Communica-
    tion, 122
Coleman, W.F., 78
Colombia
  ACPO, 81–82, 84, 90
  breastfeeding campaign, 133
  Candelaria Project, 119, 136
  coffee industry, 51
  Community Systems Foundation, 141
  education coordination, 137
  INRAVISION, 22
  Integrated Nutrition Improvement Project,
    130
  Northern Cauca Project of the Agricultural
    Institute, 62
  nutrition behavior, 102–103
  soybeans, 144–145
  weaning, 108
Contreras-Budge, E. 35, 72
Cooke, T.M., 10, 123
Coombs, Philip H., 47–51, 54, 61–62, 64,
    67, 70, 84–85
Cornell University Medical School, 120
Costa Rica
  extension activities, 50
  radio farm forum, 78–9
  radio and nutrition, 122, 132, 145
Cuba, literacy project, 19

Diffusion of Innovations, 18, 31–37, 48, 72,
    91, 161
Dodds, Tony, 7, 19, 79, 133
Dr. Hakim project. *See* Tunisia
Drake, William D., 119

East Pakistan, Allen study, 41
ECA-FAO Joint Agricultural Division, 47–50,
    60, 70
Ecuador
  agricultural program, 60

ORS project, 129
  radio and nutrition, 123
Education
  as a social good, 16
  effects of education on agricultural produc-
    tivity, 30–33
Egypt
  National Control of Diarrheal Disease
    Program, 129
  ORS project, 121, 129–130, 148
  nutrition survey, 101
Ekpere, J.A., 70–71
El Salvador
  ITV Project, 4, 21
  technology importation, 12
Esman, Milton 59
Ethiopia. *See also* ECA-FAO.
  extension activities, 50
Eveland, J., 50, 67
Evenson, Robert, 38, 44, 48, 50, 52–53
Extension Activities, 33–56, 61–72,
    117–120, 164

Fagen, Richard, 19
Farmer Education, 30–39, 43–46, 56–57
Farquhar, John, 7
Feder, Gershon, 32, 66
Feedforward, 10–11, 61–64, 83
Feeling Good television series. *See* United
    States
Fisher, J.D., 49, 51
Florida State University, 82
Foote, Dennis, 114, 123, 128, 146
Formacion, Candelaria S., 101, 108, 111,
    123, 130, 134, 137, 146
Freire, Paulo, 84
Friend, Jamesine, 6, 20, 150
Fussell and Haaland, 134

Gambia, The
  Mass Media and Health Practices Project
    (MMHP), 121, 123, 127–130, 135,
    146, 148
  Radio Gambia, 21
  rice-growing project, 57–58
  visual materials, use of, 134
Ghana, Radio Forum, 78–79
Gilmore, Judith, 139, 143
Gleason, Gary, 56
Gomez Age-Weight Classification, 107
Graham, Jack, 4
Green, James, 125, 130

Greiner, Ted, 105
Griffiths, Marcia, 110, 126, 134, 146
Guatemala
    agricultural politics, 4
    Basic Village Education (BVE) Program,
        76–78, 89, 92, 150
    community leaders training, 58
    extension activities, 34
    INCAP, 110, 112, 142
    Institute for Nutrition of Central America
        and Panama, 138–139
    Ministry of Agriculture, 4
    national out-of-school education, 22
    nutrition behavior, 102–103
    radio use, 125
Gwatkin, Davison R., 119, 138–139

Habicht, Jean-Pierre, 110, 112
Hagen, Everett, 156
Haiti, Radio Docteur, 122
Hall, Budd, 7, 19, 79, 133
Hanover Outreach Project. *See* Jamaica
Harrison, James Q., 43, 52, 65–66, 69, 85
Harvard Institute for International Develop-
    ment, 116
Hayami, Yujiro, 29, 34, 40–41, 43–44
Herdt, Robert W., 32, 34
Higgins, Margot, 122, 134
Honduras
    ACPH, 84
    Mass Media and Health Practices Project
        (MMHP), 114, 121, 123, 126–130,
        148, 150, 156–159
Hornik, Robert, 4, 123
Hudson, Heather, 9
Huffman, Wallace E., 31, 37–38
Hyman, Herbert H., 69

Imesi project. *See* Nigeria
INCAP (Incaparina). *See* Guatemala
Incentives for Educators and Clients, 143–145
India
    All India Radio, 125
    CARE, 122
    community development program, 51, 58
    consumption, 100
    extension activities, 50
    farm yields, 65, 67
    Intensive Agricultural District Program, 51
    language problems, 124
    Lele study, 41
    Narangwal study, 138

nutrition education, 138
    radio farm broadcasts, 70, 78–79
    Satellite Instructional Television Experiment
        (SITE), 8, 74–75, 84, 124
    Tamil Nadu, 108, 112, 125, 130, 136,
        145, 157
    village worker training, 54
    World Bank Training and Visit System, 66
Indian Institute of Mass Communication, 71
Indonesia
    consumption survey, 100
    nutrition education program, 121, 126–
        127, 130, 134, 143–144, 146–148
    protein needs, 112
    radio broadcasts, 137
    radio listening clubs, 80
Infant formula marketing industry, 105
Inkeles, Alex, 36
Institutions, 157–158, 161
    research institutions, 44–45, 61
International Nutrition Communication
    Service, 101
Investments
    education, 33, 45
    nutrition, 118, 145–147
Iran, Radio farm forums, 78

Jamaica, Hanover Outreach Nutrition
    Program, 119–120
Jamison, Dean, 16, 18, 33, 36–37, 83, 146,
    156
Jelliffe, Derrick B., 104–105, 130, 133
Jelliffe, Patrice, 104–105, 130, 133
Jha, Dananatha, 38
John Snow Public Health Group, 129
Jordan, nutrition behavior, 102–103
Just, R., 32

Katz, Elihu, 56
Kazunga, David K., 50, 70
Kenya. *See also* ECA-FAO
    diffusion system, 56
    extension activities, 49–51
    Kenyan Tea Development Project,
        64–65
    Tetu extension system, 56–57.
Kidd, David W., 70–72
Kislev, Yoav, 53
Klein, R.S., 112
Klees, Steven, 78
Klonglan, Gerald E., 78, 84, 86
Knudsen, Odin K., 100, 110–111

Korea
  agricultural broadcasting, 70
  CARE project, 122, 134
  extension activities, 68
  Korean Educational Development Institute,
    21
  Office of Rural Development, 70
Krishna, Raj, 40

Latin America
  extension activities, 48, 51, 53, 68
  radio schools (ACPO), 81–83
  radio use, 125
  weaning practices, 138
Lau, Lawrence, 16, 33, 36–37, 156
Lazarsfeld, Paul, 10, 56
Lee, Chin-Chuan, 125
Legitimation, 10
Lele, Uma J., 41
Lerner, Daniel, 156
Leslie, Joanne, 124
Lesotho
  nutrition survey, 101
  radio and nutrition, 124
Levine, Gene, 69
Liberia, nutrition survey, 101
Lionberger, Herbert F., 60, 62–63, 70
Lockheed, Marlaine E., 33, 35–37, 110, 156

McAnany, Emile, 4, 18, 83
McClelland, David, 154
McDermott, J.K., 11, 44
McDivitt, Judith A., 82
McDowell, Jeffrey, 41, 72
Madagascar. *See* Malagasy Republic
Magasana 99. See Philippines
Mahai, B.A.P., 133
Malagasy Republic, Extension Activities, 50.
  See also ECA-FAO
Malawi. *See also* ECA-FAO
  farmer education, 61
  information needs survey, 86
  radio listening club, 84
  radio use, 70, 72
Malaysia, farm broadcast programs, 70
Manoff, Richard K., 122–123
  Philippines campaign, 124, 146–147
Marshal Plan, x
Martorell, Reynaldo, 112
Mass Media and Health Practices Project
  (MMHP). *See* The Gambia and Honduras
Mathur, J.C., 70, 78

Maunder, Addison H., 49
Mayo, John K., 4, 69, 124–125
MEB. *See* Brazil
Melmed, Arthur, 6
Merton, Robert, 3, 10
Mexico, Plan Puebla, 22, 60, 64, 156
Micronesia, Yap Marketing Project, 140–142,
  144, 148
Mobilization, 19
Mody, Bela, 74–75
Montague, Joel, 122, 134
Morgan, Robert M., 81–82
Moris, Jon, 53–54, 65–66
Morocco
  consumption survey, 100
  food programs, 139–140, 145
  nutrition education, 101, 148
Morss, Elliott R., 47, 52–53, 57–58, 62–65,
  67, 69
Mosher, Arthur T., 43, 48–50, 53–54, 92

National Control of Diarrheal Diseases Project.
  See Egypt
Nelson, Ralph E., 31, 50, 70
Nepal
  agricultural radio programs, 69, 72
  farming systems approach, 63
  nutrition survey, 101
  Radio Nepal, 69
  radio ownership, 70
  radio use, 4, 124
Nesman, Edgar G., 32
Nestle Company, 105
Neurath, P., 78
Nicaragua
  nutrition education, 100, 123, 157
  Radio Mathematics Project, 6, 9, 20, 150
Nigeria
  agriculture and radio, 70–72
  extension saturation project, 50
  extension services, 49
  farmer's associations funds, 67
  Imesi project, 138
  radio use, 70–71
  Tiv Bams, 67, 91, 144
  tobacco company, 65
  Uboma Development project, 63
Nutrition Education
  as complement to material inputs, 137–143
  effects at the household level, 100–101
  effects within the household, 101–102
Nyerere, Julius, 133

Opoku, A.A., 78
Oral Rehydration, 113–114, 121, 128–130, 135, 142, 144, 146, 150, 163
Organizations
 agricultural, 41–42, 78–84
 local groups, 78–83
Orivel, François, 35, 44, 149
O'Sullivan, Jeremiah, 34–36, 44, 50, 78, 125, 156
Outreach Programs, 119–121, 125

Paige, Donald, 4
Pakistan, 100–101
Parker, Edwin, 9
Patel, A.U., 70–71
Pelto, Gretel H., 112
Perraton, Hilary, 9, 61, 70, 72
Peru
 nutrition behavior, 102–103
 weaning, 108
Phelps, E., 31
Philippines
 Masagana 99, 75–76, 83, 89, 92
 nutrition, 111, 123, 148
 Ruttan study, 41
Plan Puebla. *See* Mexico
Politics
 and communication projects, 5–6
 failures in projects, 24–26
 project attractiveness, 161–162
Post, James, 105
Project Design, 162–163. *See also* Channels
Promotora Program. *See* Colombia

Radio Farm Forums, 78–81, 90
Radio School Movement, 81–83
Ramadasmurthy, V., 124
Rasmuson, Mark, 122
Reutlinger, Schlomo, 97
Rice, E.B., 47–51, 53–54, 68–69
Rody, Nancy, 140–141
Rogers, Everett M., 18, 32, 35–37, 50, 67, 71–72, 78–79, 150
Roling, Niels, 44, 51, 56
Romweber, S.T., 10, 123
Rosenberg, Irwin, 111
Roy, Prodipto, 35, 78–79
Rundfunk und Fernseh and Africa Asia Bureau, 78
Rutman, Max, 138
Ruttan, Vernon W., 29, 34, 40–41, 43–44

Samoa, Television Education, 20
Sanghvi, Tina, 104, 106
Sankar, Pamela, 123
Scandizzi, Pasquale L., 100
Schramm, Wilbur, x, 6, 18, 20, 78–79, 83
Schuh, G. Edward, 44–45
Schultz, Theodore W., 15–16, 29, 32, 48, 156
Scrimshaw, Nevin S., 112
Scrimshaw, Susan, 110
Selowsky, Marcelo, 97, 110–111
Senegal. *See also* ECA-FAO
 extension activities, 51
 Radio Dissou, 11, 83
 worker training, 58
Senghor, Leopold, 83
Shepard, Donald, 146
Shingi, Prakash, 74–75
Shoemaker, Floyd, 32, 71, 150
Silberman, D., 32
SITE. *See* India
Slade, Roger, 66
Smith, David H., 36
Smith, William A., 113, 123, 127–129, 135
Social Marketing Projects, xiii, 140–142, 144
Social Network, 136, 160
Somalia, Extension Activites, 50
South Korea
 communications for development, xi
 extension activities, 50–51
Spain, Sikandra, 134
Sri Lanka
 consumption survey, 100
 nutrition survey, 101
 radio campaign for nutrition, 145
 radio use, 122
Stanford Heart Disease Prevention Program, 7
Stockley, Trevor L., 70, 73–74
Suchman, Edward A., 14
Svenning, Lynne, 36, 72
Swaziland
 farming systems approach, 63
 ORS project, 121, 123, 128, 148

Taiwan
 agriculture, 57, 63, 70
 communication for development, xi
 farm information systems, 60, 62, 65, 144
 field organization, 91
Tamil Nadu. *See* India

Tanzania
  Food is Life Campaign, 133
  Man is Health Campaign, 133, 145
  mobilization strategy, 19, 133
  nutrition education, 101, 133, 145, 148
  Nyerere, Julius, 133
  radio and adult education, 7
  TANU political party, 133
Thailand
  Behrman study, 41
  nutrition, 102, 119–120
Thorat, Sudhakar, 43–44, 50, 55, 60, 69
Tiv Bams. *See* Nigeria
Tollini, Helio, 44–45
Toquero, Zenaida, 40
Training and Visit System. *See* World Bank
Tunisia
  Dr. Hakim project, 123
  nutrition, 102–103
  weaning, 108
Turkey, farm yields, 65, 67

Uganda, Agriculture, 70. *See also* ECA-FAO
UN agencies, 165
UNESCO, Radio forums, 78
United States
  extension activities, 44, 51
  Feeling Good television series, 124
University of North Carolina School of Public
    Health, 141
University of the West Indies, 120
USAID, 97, 163
  Bolivia, 141
  Guatemala, 4, 76
  Mass Media and Health Practices Project
    (MMHP), 127
  Nigeria, 50

Valdivia, Margaret, 104, 132–133, 137
Van der Vynckt, Susan, 132
Van Esterik, Penny, 105
Vemury, Merlyn, 102, 104, 108, 114
Village Extension Worker (VEW), 65–66
Viravaidhya, Khun Vina, 119, 121

Waisanen, F.B., 35, 78–79
Wall Street Journal, 105
Weaning, 107–113
Welch, Finis, 16, 30–31
Wharton, Clifton R. Jr., 31–32
White, Robert A., 67, 81
Winikoff, Beverly, 104
Wise, Robert P., 142
Wolfe, Barbara, 16, 100, 157
World Bank, 29, 97–98, 100, 165
  extension activities, 50
  The Gambia, 57
  Indonesia, 121, 126
  Tamil Nadu in India, 130
  training and visit system, 65–66, 85, 89,
    151
World Health Organization (WHO), 105, 128
Wright, Charles, 69
Wright, Maria da Gloria Miotto, 141

Yap District Health Department. *See* Microne-
    sia

Zaire, Nutrition, 111, 120, 132
Zambia. *See also* ECA-FAO
  extension activities, 50
  radio farm forums, 78
Zeitlin, Marian, 101, 108, 111–112, 123,
    130, 134, 137, 146